Memories After Abortion

Edited by

Vivian Wahlberg

Professor Emeritus
Nordic School of Public Health, Göteborg
Registered Nurse and Midwife
Doctor of Medical Science

Foreword by

Ann Thomson

Radcliffe Publishing
Oxford ● Seattle

Radcliffe Publishing Ltd
18 Marcham Road
Abingdon
Oxon OX14 1AA
United Kingdom

www.radcliffe-oxford.com
Electronic catalogue and worldwide online ordering facility.

———————————————————————

British Library Cataloguing in Publication Data

A catalogue record for this book is available from the British Library.

ISBN-10: 1 84619 131 9
ISBN-13: 978 1 84619 131 2

Typeset by Aarontype Ltd, Easton, Bristol
Printed and bound by TJ International Ltd, Padstow, Cornwall

After my abortion I dreamt one night that my little baby flew away on a wing – further and further out into the universe, and I felt a great sense of relief ... but thought that one day my baby will surely come back to me again ...

Anna-Carin

Contents

Foreword

Consideration of abortion causes a lot of distress, anxiety and debate within society. This is because it is inextricably linked with society's views of life and sexuality. It is also because the word 'abortion' is frequently linked with illegality and being undertaken in 'back streets'. There is evidence that women have been aware of methods of obtaining the end of a pregnancy for centuries. Currently, the WHO estimate that 20 million abortions are carried out illegally in the world and illicit, illegal abortion is a major cause of maternal mortality. This is a disaster for the whole of society, but in particular for families and the women.

This book was originally published in Swedish and reports on research carried out with women who have had legal abortions, recently and in the past, with the partners of those women, with women in both Sweden and Italy and with priests and psychiatrists who have had experience of counselling women who have had an abortion. There is a perception in society that girls and women requesting abortion are immoral, irresponsible and sexually incontinent. However, the findings reported here show how women, and men, do not approach abortion lightly and the consequences, both physical and psychological, vividly portrayed in their memories of the baby they have lost, can stay with them for many years. Many report of the tragedy of the situation they find themselves in and of the need to ensure that contraception is available and accessible to all.

The translation of this book into English means that it is now available to a wider audience. The issues can be debated throughout the English-speaking world and the 'Epilogue' discussing the ethical issues of abortion will enhance that debate. This book should be read by young people and their teachers so that the issues around sexuality and the use of contraception can be fully explored. It should be read by women and men so that they can debate and understand each others' views and experiences in their relationships. It should be read by nurses, midwives, doctors, health-service administrators and those providing social care so that, hopefully, those who need an abortion can be provided with safe care, both physically and psychologically. In order to prevent the tragedy of an unwanted pregnancy, effective, appropriate and accessible contraceptive facilities must be provided to all who want to use them. This book adds to the literature demonstrating the needs for these facilities worldwide.

Ann M Thomson
Professor of Midwifery
School of Nursing, Midwifery and Social Work
University of Manchester
September 2006

Foreword to the Swedish edition

Today, about 34 000 women per year have an abortion in Sweden. One may ask why this happens in such a small country as Sweden with sex education as a compulsory school subject, with outpatient clinics for adolescents and with free access to a number of different contraceptives. For me, the woman's right to decide upon her own reproduction is a fundamental human right, of which legal abortion is an important part. To be able to preserve the right to free abortion, but also to decrease the risk of unintentional pregnancies, it is important to understand what factors underlie a decision to have an abortion.

In this book *Memories After Abortion*, with Vivian Wahlberg as the main author, women and men describe their experiences of going through this procedure. A decision to undergo an abortion is never an easy one and the subsequent memories remain throughout life. It is also clear from the related experiences how important it is for the woman to get help and support. At the same time abortion may be seen as the only possible solution to the situation at hand. The environment we live in certainly plays a major role in the attitude towards sexuality and abortion. It is therefore important to obtain information about how young people themselves – not only in Sweden, but also in another country such as Italy – look upon these questions.

The book also gives broad information about how not only the view of abortion but also the wording of the Abortion Act has changed over time since the beginning of the twentieth century. As a midwife, Vivian Wahlberg has experiences herself from abortions and deliveries and has also carried out research within this field. All this has resulted in a book filled with young people's thoughts and feelings, as well as relevant facts essential for an objective discussion of the right to free abortion. Thus there are very good reasons why this book fulfils the main author's hopes of elucidating and increasing the understanding of the abortion problem and of stimulating further discussion and reflection.

Marc Bygdeman
Professor Emeritus
Karolinska Institute
Stockholm
December 2005

Preface

Once again abortion is a highly topical issue after several reports of an increase in abortion rates, especially among teenagers. During the seven-year period from 1995 to 2002, the number of teenage abortions in Sweden increased by nearly 50%, despite the fact that contraceptives have been readily available for many decades and that 'morning-after pills' for emergency contraception can be bought without prescription at pharmacies or obtained free of charge at most of the Outpatient Clinics for Adolescents in Sweden.

In Sweden a new Abortion Act came into force in January 1975, which protects women from illegal and dangerous abortions carried out by inexperienced and unqualified individuals. It is also important to protect the woman's sense of well-being, so that abortion is only performed as a last resort. No one wishes to have an unplanned pregnancy – this is evident from the narratives presented in this book. Both girls and boys describe their experiences when the unexpected happens to them – how everything turns into darkness and confusion when they are far too young to become parents and do not want a child, or else they do not want a child just now or with this partner. It is a source of physical and mental stress as everything in their life seems to be going wrong at once.

This book sheds light on the reality of how a human being is formed from the most minute particle, the *zygote*, at the moment of fertilisation. This develops into an *embryo* (a multi-celled body), which then gives rise to the *fetus* and finally the *child*. The various developmental stages of the fetus and its size at weeks 1, 8, 12, etc. are also briefly discussed.

In addition, the book considers some religious and cultural differences in attitudes to abortion, the Abortion Act in Sweden, contraception and the morning-after pill, the attitudes of young people to abortion and sexual relationships, and their own narratives about unwanted pregnancy. Some older women also describe their memories of abortion that they underwent many years ago.

The narratives in this book almost universally refer to the so-called *early abortions*, which are performed before the end of week 12 of pregnancy. However, some abortions are performed much later. In Sweden, abortion is freely available up to the end of week 18 of pregnancy. If the pregnancy has progressed beyond week 18, an abortion may only be performed if it can be demonstrated that there are special reasons for the procedure, and following an evaluation by the Swedish National Board of Health and Welfare. However, an abortion may never be performed so late that the fetus is judged to be capable of surviving outside the woman's body.

The book also describes the personal experiences of psychiatrists and Catholic priests, summarised from conversational therapy with or confessions of women after abortions, which in many cases were performed several decades earlier. Some of these women had never spoken to anyone about the abortion before, but had carried their memories and pain alone as a dark shadow hanging over their lives. This illustrates the importance of being able to talk about issues such as the experience of abortion in order to be able to leave the issues behind and move on with one's life.

I shall end this introduction by quoting some words after an abortion. It derives from the dream of a young girl, who shortly after her abortion told me:

> ... After my abortion I dreamt one night that my little baby flew away on a wing – further and further out into the universe, and I felt a great sense of relief ... but thought that one day my baby will surely come back to me again ...

It is quite common for women who have experienced abortion to talk in metaphors and symbols, which can sometimes be almost poetical.

Recently I found an article by the author and poet Ylva Eggehorn in a Swedish newspaper. It had the title 'Poetry carries a reality', and among other things it discussed the complexity and mystery of faith and life, painful experiences, and mutual understanding in harmony. At the beginning of the article there is an illustration of a baby on a swan wing, and the article ends as follows:

> Why bury a child on a wing of a swan, as they did in Denmark about 10 000 years ago? Is this 'just poetry'? What then is 'poetry'? Something which 'does not exist' or something which carries a reality? Our mission should then be to find out and formulate what this reality consists of, and the nature of its distinctive character. The human being exists. The body exists. The movements exist ...
>
> What in fact is happening when we place a child, who has recently died, on the wing of a swan before we bury it? What happens in that movement, in the moment when we place it there? Why do tears come into my eyes when I think about it? Where does the feeling of relief come from ... ?

The author continues 'I think more and more about what it would imply if we really could find a language that could describe the whole complexity and joy of life ...'

Much of this book deals with the complexity of life, but also with pleasure, joy and relief at different levels and in different situations. Dreams and metaphors are often used to describe something that is difficult to express by other means. For instance, a woman spoke about a 'special trauma' that had occurred 12–15 years earlier. She went backwards and forwards in time, using different metaphors for the trauma and describing how it had negatively influenced her life, until suddenly she mentioned the word 'abortion.' It was like peeling an onion, removing layer after layer of repressed sadness and despair until she eventually reached the innermost part of the core and cried out 'Now, at last, I am free!'

In this book, young people's narratives describe crossroads in life, risk-taking behaviour, difficult decisions, guilt and responsibility, fiction and escape, different lifestyles and the inexorable power of the past over the present.

It is my hope that this book will help both to increase the reader's understanding of the abortion problem and to encourage more discussion and reflection on this complex issue.

Vivian Wahlberg
Stockholm
September 2006

About the editor

Vivian Wahlberg graduated as Doctor of Medical Science at the Karolinska Institute, Stockholm, in 1982. Her thesis was entitled *'Reconsideration of Credé Prophylaxis.* A Study of Maternity and Neonatal Care.'* She is a registered nurse and midwife, and has a Bachelors degree in sociology and behavioural science.

She was made a Visiting Professor at the University of Calgary in 1983, was awarded an International Professorship at the University of California, San Francisco in 1986, was a Visiting Professor/Project Leader (part-time) at the University of Colombia, South America from 1985 to 1987, and was made Doctor Honoris Causa in law at the University of Calgary in 1985.

She is now Professor Emeritus at the Nordic School of Public Health, Göteborg, Sweden, where she held a professorship from 1987 to 1999. She is a frequent keynote speaker and research collaborator both nationally and internationally in the fields of public health, maternity and neonatal healthcare, adoption, abortion issues, etc.

---

* Silver nitrate prophylaxis against gonococcal ophthalmia (infection in children's eyes).

About the contributors

António Barbosa da Silva was born on the Cape Verde Islands. He pursued his academic studies in Portugal, Norway and Sweden, and received his doctorate in theology from the University of Uppsala, Sweden, in 1982. His doctorate thesis was entitled *'Phenomenology of Religion as a Philosophical Problem.'* He became Associate Professor in Philosophy of Religion at the University of Uppsala in 1993, and from 1993 to 1995 he was an adjunct Professor of Philosophy of Sciences and Healthcare Ethics at the Nordic School of Public Health, Göteborg, Sweden.

In 1995 he was appointed Professor of Philosophy of Sciences and Systematic Theology in Norway. He is now Professor of Ethics and Philosophy of Sciences at the University of Stavanger, Norway. He is a highly respected lecturer on the international circuit, and is the author of several works on the inter-religious dialogue of systematic theology, healthcare ethics, etc.

Marianne Bengtsson Agostino graduated as Doctor of Public Health in 1992 from the Nordic School of Public Health, Göteborg, Sweden, with a thesis entitled *'Cultural, Social and Individual Aspects of Abortion. A Comparative Study in Italy and Sweden.'* She is a registered nurse, has a BSc in sociology, and has extensive experience of education and research in paediatric healthcare, anthropology and a variety of public welfare issues.

For several years she has taught advanced nursing courses at the University of Rome, the Red Cross University College of Nursing, Stockholm, and the Università Campus Bio-Medico, Rome. She has also translated many books from Italian into Swedish.

Lars I Holmberg, MD, is a paediatrician and Head of the Child Health Unit in the County of Dalarna, Sweden. In 2003 he gained an MSc in public health from the Nordic School of Public Health, Göteborg. His thesis was entitled *'Young Men and Unplanned Pregnancy. Risk Behaviour and Need for Support.'*

He has extensive experience of working in paediatric clinics and school health services, and since 1984 he has worked at the Borlänge Outpatient Clinic for Adolescents, Sweden. His research interests include public health, unhealthy behaviour and risk-taking behaviour among teenagers, and health services for adolescents, particularly for young men.

Chapter 1

What in fact is a human being?

Vivian Wahlberg

Introduction

The purpose of this chapter is to describe briefly how attitudes to abortion, from both cultural and religious perspectives, have changed over time, and to outline the development of the fetus during the various stages of pregnancy. Also described is a clinical experience in the 1950s which has remained in the author's memory as an example of a situation specifically related to abortion.

A brief history of attitudes to the fetus and abortion

The early scriptures

Historically, and in different religions, there have been many different views and opinions about the child, both before and after birth.[1] In writings from China, abortion was mentioned around 4700 years ago. In ancient Greece, a few hundred years before Christ, Plato and Aristotle advocated abortion for hereditary reasons, and also stated that women should not give birth after the ideal age for childbirth. Furthermore, abortion was to be used to limit the number of children born in order to maintain the ideal nation.

Accordingly, in ancient Greece abortion was defended as a necessary method of limiting the growth of the population. During the same period the women of Rome used various forms of contraception, but nevertheless abortions frequently occurred. Infanticide was even more common than abortion in Roman times. In ancient Egypt there were burial ceremonies for aborted fetuses but not for stillborn children.

Remarkably, in the older European literature it was recommended that abortions should take place as late as possible, one stated reason being that this would lead to less dramatic complications for the woman.

There is no mention of abortion in the Bible, but in some of the older Jewish writings there is indirect evidence of opposition to abortion on the grounds that life is a gift from God. There is written evidence that during the first centuries AD the Apostolic Fathers condemned the termination of pregnancy.[2,3]

The development of the fetus

Ideas about the different stages of fetal development and views as to whether the fetus has any real value or a soul have varied from culture to culture. For at least

2000 years different theories have prevailed about the stages of development of the fetus and of the soul from vegetative to animal and ultimately to a rational, intelligent being.

The great philosophers, including Aristotle (384–322 BC), Dante (1265–1321), Thomas Aquinas (1225–1274) and others,[4,5] have discussed the development of the fetus from a shapeless fluid (Latin *non-formatus*) to a being with a sensitive soul that finally, after 40–50 days, attains human status (Latin *formatus et animatus),* when the extremities can be discerned. In this final stage the fetus was considered to be a rational, intellectual being (Latin *formatus intellectiva*). Aristotle believed that when the fetus had become 'human-like' it had an intellectual soul.[4,6]

Even today, in many countries and in many cultures and religions the question arises as to when the fertilised egg actually has the potential to be a human life with human dignity that should be inviolable and treated with respect.

Some definitions of abortion (see also *Chapter 2)*

- Abortion is defined as termination of a pregnancy by removal or delivery of the fetus. The word abortion comes from the Latin word *'abortio',* meaning untimely birth.
- Spontaneous abortion is commonly referred to as miscarriage.
- Induced abortion is an abortion induced by either medicinal means or surgical intervention.
- Early abortion is an abortion that takes place before the end of week 12 of pregnancy.
- Late abortion is an abortion that takes place after the beginning of week 13 of pregnancy.

Attitudes of different religions to contraception and abortion

With the advance of Christianity, views on abortion and contraception changed, and around AD 300 abortion was forbidden. It was considered that the fertilised egg should have the right to full human dignity from the moment of conception. Abortion was regarded as equivalent to infanticide, and could not be reconciled with the Christian teaching that 'thou shall not kill.'[1]

The middle of the fourteenth century saw the beginning of the persecution of women and men who had sufficient knowledge of medicine, contraceptive methods and childbirth to enable them to perform abortions. Even in our own time – for example, in certain states in the USA – there are strong reactionary forces against abortion, and persecution and attempted murder of those who have performed or assisted with abortions have been documented up to the late twentieth century.

In general it may be said that virtually all countries and religions have respect for the humanity of the unborn child, but that attitudes towards contraception and abortion vary widely from one religion to another.

The Catholic Church

Catholicism is the largest Christian denomination in the world, with 900 million baptised members. In Sweden there are about 165 000 Catholics.[7] The Catholic

Church regards contraception as a sin and believes that there is potential for a human life from the moment of conception, and that this should not be violated.

According to the teachings of the Catholic Church, the right to contraception and self-determination must never be practised at the cost of the right to life of another human being. Every human life is sacred and thereby sacrosanct. Even if the fetus is at an early stage of development, it is an evolving human being, and for this reason the Catholic Church regards abortion as murder. Abortion is only acceptable if the mother's life is in danger.

The Protestant Church

In the year 2002 the Protestant Church in Sweden had just over seven million members. It has a considerably more liberal view now than in earlier times, and officially permits abortion even though this is at the cost of the life of the fetus. A more liberal and positive view of sexuality and contraception has developed since the later part of the twentieth century. Sexual relationships before marriage, as well as abortion, divorce and remarriage, are accepted by the Protestant Church.

In 1975 a new law relating to abortion was introduced in Sweden, which in practice means that women have a legal right to abortion up to the end of week 18 of pregnancy. If there is a particularly strong reason for doing so, an abortion may be performed after weeks 18–20 of pregnancy, when permission has been granted by the National Board of Health and Welfare,[8] and on rare occasions even later, although this situation has been widely criticised.

Judaism

There are about 20 000 Jewish people living in Sweden.[7] According to Jewish belief it is a religious duty to be married and a 'divine gift' to be fertile and prolific.[9] A Jew should practise sexual activity and endeavour to have at least two children, a situation which is common within the Jewish tradition.

Jewish belief does not recognise the fetus as an independent being while it remains in the mother's womb. However, the unborn life is to be safeguarded, in principle because according to the scriptures human beings should 'multiply and fill the earth.' According to the *Talmud* (the Jewish scriptures) the fetus is 'pure liquid' for the first 40 days, and only on the fortieth day does it become a true fetus.[9] The individual human life is considered to begin at birth. Thus because the fetus is not perceived to be a person until birth, an abortion cannot be regarded as murder.

Nevertheless, Jews have strict views on abortion and believe that the unborn life must be safeguarded. However, according to a more liberal attitude that also prevails, abortion may be permitted not only when the mother's life is in danger, but also in other specific circumstances, such as mental disorder/illness.

Islam: the Muslim faith

Islam is the second largest religion in Sweden.[7] In 1999 it was calculated that there were around 250 000 Muslim immigrants in Sweden.

Islam is a religion with a strong focus on social issues, marriage and the family. Sexuality is seen as a very important part of the relationship between husband and wife. Family planning and contraception are regarded by certain Muslims as being in conflict with the Koran, which emphasises the duty or blessing of producing offspring. Questions concerning abortion are considered to be very complex and are the subject of much controversy. However, it is generally believed that abortion should not be permitted after 120 days' pregnancy, unless it is necessary in order to save the mother's life. According to Muslim tradition the fetus is a living being after day 120, and abortion is therefore forbidden after that stage.[9]

Hinduism and Buddhism

It is estimated that around 6000 Hindus and 15 000 Buddhists are living in Sweden today.[7] Some Hindus and Buddhists believe that the unborn fetus and the mother giving birth are unclean. There are also different views as to when the fetus or child 'belongs to the earth and humanity.'[10] For example, Indonesian Hindus consider that until the child is 7 months old its soul is part of the universe, divine and unspoilt, and has not yet been formed into a separate individual. Both local and national customs reflect different opinions and different rules. In general it is believed that one should never take or harm a life, and usually there is a reprimand or some kind of penalty following an abortion.

Thus within every religion there is a variety of viewpoints and arguments relating to sexuality, contraception, abortion and the human value of the unborn child.

From zygote to embryo to fetus to child

Medico-technological advances and the development of new medical specialties have led to rapid progress in the fields of fertility and neonatal research. From the moment of fertilisation a new human being starts to take shape, but when exactly does human life begin? And at what precise stage of development does the fetus acquire human value? Development occurs along a continuum from the *zygote* (the fertilised egg cell, weeks 0–1) to the *embryo* (the multi-celled body that develops from the zygote, weeks 1–8), the *fetus* (weeks 8–28) and finally the *child* (from the moment of birth, or when the fetus has reached week 28 of the pregnancy or shows clear signs of life at birth).

Human dignity and our view of man

Our views on human value in relation to the fetus depend to a large extent on whether our worldview of man is scientific, existential or humanistic. They also depend on how we define the word 'value', which may refer to any of the following:

- the human value of the fetus/unborn child itself
- the human value of the fetus/unborn child to the parents
- the value of the tissues from the aborted fetus for treatment and/or transplantation in conditions such as Parkinson's disease, diabetes mellitus, etc.

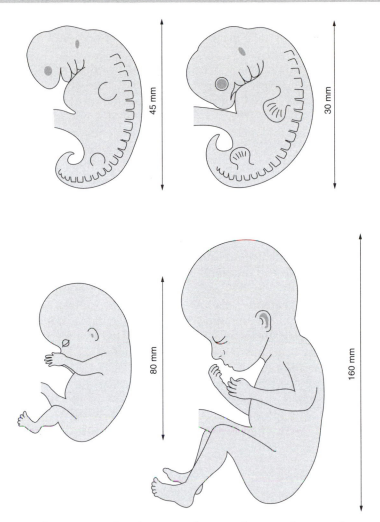

Figure 1.1   The various developmental stages from embryo to fetus.
Illustrator: Lena Lyons.

If we go back to the earliest stages, namely the zygote or embryo, as for instance
with *in-vitro* fertilisation, do we see the fertilised egg or the deep-frozen embryo
only as potential for human life, or do we see it as a useful source of stem cells, or
even as having a direct profit value? Where and when along this continuum from
conception to birth is the point at which the unborn child acquires human value?
These are questions that we must reflect on today.

Some reflections on the capabilities of the fetus

It has long been known that from as early as week 6 of pregnancy the fetal brain
begins to function so well that an electroencephalogram (EEG) can be recorded,
and the fetal heart is beating. By 8 weeks the fetus is able to grip an object, and if
the object is sharp and stinging, it will quickly withdraw its hand.[11]

More than 90% of the abortions that take place in Sweden occur before week 12 of pregnancy, but many take place up to week 18 of pregnancy, and in some cases even later.

A research poll on public opinion conducted in Sweden in 1992, in which around 1000 individuals were questioned, revealed that 88% of respondents considered that 12 weeks should normally be the latest time at which an abortion is performed. Only 4% considered that it could be performed after 12 weeks.

There have been major developments in research and changes in attitude during the 14 years or so since that opinion poll was published. We now have further evidence of the early capabilities of the fetus, and this has evoked greater respect for and demands for the protection of the unborn child.

Borderline cases for the ethically acceptable

By virtue of advances in medico-technological development, we are now able to keep a fetus alive outside the mother's body at increasingly earlier stages of its life. Infants weighing only 500–600 grams at birth, and sometimes even less, can now survive. In recent years in the USA, where large resources are set aside for research on these issues, several specific cases have attracted attention. For instance, there have been births as early as weeks 21–23 of pregnancy. Among those cases that it has been possible to follow up, many of these children have developed without serious adverse effects.[12]

These examples may be considered in light of the fact that in several parts of the world it is permissible to perform abortion up to week 24 of pregnancy. Has the limit of what is ethically acceptable therefore been overstepped? And when very late abortions are performed, is the human dignity of the unborn child being violated?

A personal experience from the 1950s

So close to life ...

For me the abortion issue has been a reality since the time when, as a young midwifery student in the 1950s, I had a confusing experience in a gynaecological operating theatre. For several weeks I had been doing my practical training on the delivery ward, and had had many exciting moments and experiences in delivery care. I considered it a great privilege to be able to work so close to life, and I was filled with wonder and joy each time I was able to help a new person into the world. To be able to share this miracle with the happy parents made me certain that my choice of career was the right one.

But then came my move to the gynaecological department. My main assignment there during the first week was to assist with abortions. The patients ranged from very young girls to mature women, who for different and apparently understandable reasons had been forced to choose an abortion as the only possible solution to their situation. Nearly all of these abortions took place before week 12 of pregnancy. The atmosphere on the ward was friendly and tolerant, and the patients were cared for with respect and understanding.

During my second week on the gynaecological ward I had to assist in the department where more advanced gynaecological operations took place. On the operating list there were several late abortions. The first one, an abortion in week 19 of pregnancy, was fairly undramatic. The next abortion was in week 22 (for a woman with a serious socio-medical problem), and the operation was performed through an abdominal incision. I vividly remember the moment when the doctor lifted out the whimpering baby and put it into a receptacle, which he then passed to me with instructions to put it in the fridge. Often I would go to the fridge and open the door slightly, full of wonder and feelings of ambivalence towards the tiny baby – who was later collected with the rest of the department's 'biological waste.'

The following week I returned to practice and training on the delivery ward. My first patient there was a woman who was about to give birth to a child with an expected club foot. It was to be a breech delivery, and I was fully prepared for the fact that there would be an abnormality. In fact both feet were deformed and even the child's head was deformed, and much of the brain was missing.

My clinical teacher had instructed me to immediately follow all of the resuscitation procedures necessary. A paediatrician was called in, oxygen was connected up, alternating hot and cold baths for the infant were prepared, and so on.

Once again I felt great ambivalence. How can one make such a distinction between children? The first was taken out far too early – an apparently perfect and clearly viable little human being – and was then ignored. The other, born at full term, had such severe defects that any life-supporting measures were doomed to failure. Despite this, every possible resource was used to save this gravely ill and badly deformed child, but not the other healthy, living fetus.

Ever since that time I have tried to answer the question 'What in fact is a human being?'

References

1 Trost A-C. *Abortion and Mental Difficulties* (Swedish text). Västerås: International Library, 1982.
2 Roberts A & Donaldson J. *The Anti-Nicene Fathers*. Edinburgh: WMB Eerdmans Publishing Company, 1989.
3 Andres O. *The Apostolic Fathers* (Swedish text). Stockholm: Verbum, 1992.
4 Dunstan GR & Seller MJ (eds). *The Status of the Human Embryo. Perspectives from moral tradition.* London: Oxford University Press, 1988.
5 Kjessler B. Embryo research – an ethical abomination or a chance for humanity? (Swedish text). *Läkartidningen.* 1989; **86:** 1610–13.
6 Dahlström G. The human embryo's status in the history of ideas – incorrect translations of the Bible affect the debate on abortion (Swedish text). *Läkartidningen.* 1989; **86:** 635–6.
7 Sjögren PA (ed.) *The National Encyclopaedia, Sweden* (Swedish text). Stockholm: Bra Böcker, 1997.
8 *The Swedish Abortion Act* (SFS = Svensk Författningssamling) The Swedish statute book 1974: 595 (Swedish text).
9 Görman U. Religion, sexuality and abortion. In: A-L Pehrsson (ed.) *Experiences and Personal Choices. A book on abortion* (Swedish text). Stockholm: Gothia Publishing House, 2000.

10 Einhorn L. The mystery of the ego (Swedish text). In: SVT 2, Swedish Television Channel 2 summer programme: Vetenskapens Värld *(The World of Science)*, 11 August 2003.

11 Valman HB & Pearson JF. What the fetus feels. *BMJ.* 1980; **280**: 233–4.

12 Tillander U, Larsson R, Jonsson G *et al.* It is about ethics and respect for life (Swedish text). *Svenska Dagbladet*, 6 February 1993.

Chapter 2

The abortion situation in Sweden

Vivian Wahlberg

Introduction

This chapter gives a picture of the situation with regard to abortion in Sweden, and includes a discussion of different definitions of abortion, together with a brief history of the development of this issue from the thirteenth century to the present day. In addition, various aspects of the media debate on abortion and discussions on selective abortion are summarised, and some statistical information from both Sweden and other parts of the world is presented. Different types of interventions for early and late abortions are described, and the dilemma that abortion presents for the mother and father, doctors, nurses and others is discussed. It is clear that the right to abortion is here to stay!

Different definitions of abortion

From the Latin word 'abortio'

After having an abortion, a woman may find herself with a doctor's certificate in her hand, wondering exactly what her diagnosis is and what all the Latin words mean. A few of the Latin words used in this context, and their meaning, are therefore described below.

According to the Swedish Academy's *Dictionary of the Swedish Language*,[1] the word 'abort' (or 'abortion') refers to termination of a pregnancy, or (medical) miscarriage. The word 'abortion' comes from the Latin *'abortio'*, meaning to give birth too early, to be lost, to be killed, or to die prematurely (spontaneous or induced miscarriage). Older Latin terms include *'abortus artificialis'* and *'abortus provocatus'*, both of which refer to an induced miscarriage or the artificial removal of a fetus.

The Latin term *'abortus incompletus'* means an incomplete miscarriage with part of the placenta and/or the endometrium remaining in the uterus.

Medical and daily usage of the term 'abortion'

In medical terminology the word 'abortion' is often used to cover all forms of miscarriage, spontaneous as well as induced. However, in everyday language it is most commonly used to describe a deliberately induced termination of a pregnancy before the fetus has developed to a stage at which it can be considered capable of survival outside the mother's body.

The Swedish abortion laws

The old provincial laws

For a long time abortion was forbidden in Sweden. Abortion was mentioned in the early provincial laws, and in the thirteenth century all forms of induced miscarriage were prohibited in accordance with the Västgöta law. In the fifteenth century anyone found guilty of performing an abortion faced severe punishment, and by the seventeenth century those found guilty could face the death penalty.

In the Swedish penal code of 1734 the death penalty was prescribed for any woman who had had an abortion or anyone who 'in any way advised or assisted.' Throughout Europe, right up until the nineteenth century, women who were found to have knowledge about birth control and induced miscarriage could be burnt at the stake. Just over 100 years later the punishment was reduced to flogging, forced labour, being sent to a house of correction or a maximum of six years' imprisonment. In 1921, the year when women in Sweden gained the right to vote, the punishment for those who had performed an abortion was reduced to between six months' and two years' imprisonment or penal servitude.

Illegal abortion

During the First World War and the post-war period, the number of illegal abortions in Sweden increased, and as a result more and more women had to seek hospital care for infections resulting from these illegal procedures. It was estimated that 10 000–20 000 women in Sweden had an illegal abortion each year. Those women who were found to have had an illegal abortion were punished with a one-year conditional sentence, and for the person who performed the abortion the penalty was, as mentioned above, up to two years' imprisonment or forced labour. Both men and women offered these abortion services. Two names mentioned were 'The Unskilled Labourer Eriksson in Stockholm' and 'Red Karin in Hagalund' (another part of Stockholm). For the women involved, this was a time of great uncertainty, fear, guilt and shame. Poor women also paid a high price to be rid of their unplanned pregnancy. Poison drinks and potions, knitting needles and the like were used, often resulting in serious infections that sometimes led to death.

By the late 1930s, the situation in Stockholm had become so difficult that the authorities opened a special clinic, the so-called 'Yellow Clinic' at the Sabbatsberg Hospital, specifically for women who had undergone an illegal abortion.

When the Karolinska Hospital was opened in Stockholm in 1940, one of the wards in the gynaecological department was constantly filled with women seeking help for serious infections following an illegal abortion. These complications often resulted in permanent inability to have children, and in some cases led to the woman's death.

The 1934 Abortion Committee: the first step towards legal abortion

In 1934 the Swedish government appointed a committee to investigate whether or not abortion should be permitted by law in specific cases. This investigation formed the basis of Sweden's first Abortion Act, which came into force in 1938.[2] This Act permitted abortion on the following three grounds:

- medico-social
- humanitarian
- eugenic.

Abortion on medico-social grounds was based on illness, bodily dysfunction or weakness of the woman of such a degree that the birth of the child would present a serious threat to the woman's life and health. Abortion on humanitarian grounds basically applied following incest or rape, or if the woman had not yet reached the age of 15 years. Abortion on eugenic grounds was intended to prevent the mother or father from transferring a hereditary defect that could cause mental disease, mental deficiency or other serious illnesses or deformities in the child.

New and more liberal steps

In 1946, new medico-social grounds were added.[3] A woman no longer needed to show signs of illness or weakness either when she sought an abortion or at the time of the abortion. However, it could be assumed from her living conditions and general circumstances that her physical or mental strength might be seriously impaired if she gave birth and became responsible for a child.

In the early 1960s, thousands of Swedish women with unwanted pregnancies travelled to Poland in order to have an abortion there, as the Polish law on abortion was much more liberal. This situation gave rise to considerable debate in Sweden, and the Swedish politicians appointed a new commission to investigate the subject.

During the 1960s there were successive changes in society as views not only on sexuality but also on abortion became more liberal. As a result, an increased number of applications for abortion were approved, and the number of legal abortions increased considerably. The thalidomide disaster in 1963 resulted in a new set of grounds for approval of abortion, namely when there is a risk of the child becoming ill or harmed due to a cause other than hereditary factors.[4]

A new abortion law in 1975

The present legislation on abortion in Sweden was introduced in 1974 and came into force in January 1975.[5] This new Abortion Act abrogated the former stipulations in the penal code and the previous regulation, according to which two doctors or the Swedish National Board of Health and Welfare should decide whether or not a woman should be granted permission to have an abortion. A woman now has the legal right to have an abortion up to the end of week 18 of pregnancy, after she has consulted and been examined by a doctor, who must determine the length of the pregnancy, the woman's general gynaecological state of health and any contraindications to an abortion. The doctor must also inform the woman about the different methods of abortion available and what complications might possibly occur.[6] In addition, the woman should be offered counselling both before and after the abortion.

In 1995, some changes and additions to the 1975 Abortion Act were made. Among other things it was stated that all women were granted the right to have contact with a social welfare officer, irrespective of the length of their pregnancy. Furthermore, the law was changed so that in the case of a viable fetus an abortion can no longer be permitted if the woman's life or health is in danger. Instead the concept of *prematurely induced birth* was introduced. The difference between abortion and termination of pregnancy is that an abortion has the aim of killing the fetus, whereas the aim of termination of pregnancy is the survival of both mother and child. The situation then becomes one of a prematurely induced birth. In most cases this resolves at least one problem. For example, a woman with a serious heart condition who is unable to complete her pregnancy for that reason would certainly wish her baby to survive. On the other hand, a problem may arise if a woman who is beyond week 22 of pregnancy is so desperate that she threatens to take her own life if she is not granted an abortion. In such a case her request cannot be fulfilled.

Thus, with certain reservations, every woman now has the right to have an abortion, and she does not need to explain her reasons or argue her case. However, the operation may not be performed if it is considered that it may present a serious risk to the woman's life or health. If the pregnancy has progressed beyond week 18, an abortion may only be performed if special criteria can be satisfied and the Swedish National Board of Health and Welfare has granted permission. In addition, the woman will need to have consulted a social welfare officer, who then submits a written report on the woman's current situation to the National Board of Health and Welfare. The Swedish legislation relating to abortion is only valid for women who have Swedish citizenship or who are residents in the country, a situation which is now widely criticised. However, the National Board of Health and Welfare may give their permission for a foreign national to have an abortion in Sweden if there are special reasons for this. Refugees and immigrants who are in Sweden awaiting residence permits may also be granted permission to have an abortion. However, the legislation in Sweden does not support the idea of special arrangements being made for women from other countries who wish to come to Sweden in order to have an abortion.

Debate on late abortions and abortion registers

In Sweden, the Legal Aid Council at the National Board of Health and Welfare is the authority responsible for evaluating cases where a woman is seeking an abortion that will take place after week 18 of pregnancy. The requirements for granting a request for an abortion as late as this are that there are special reasons and that the fetus is judged to be non-viable. The Legal Aid Council consists of lawyers, psychiatrists, gynaecologists and social welfare officers, as well as representatives of the National Board of Health and Welfare and the political parties.

The Council's decision is based partly on the medical and gynaecological evaluation that has been made by a gynaecologist at the clinic where the woman applied for an abortion, and partly on the social welfare officer's report. The gynaecologist's report must state clearly whether or not the fetus can be judged to be viable. Over the years it has only been in certain isolated cases that the Council has held a different opinion about the viability of a fetus from that of the gynaecologist at the clinic where the woman applied for an abortion.

In debate articles published since the late 1990s it has been suggested that it is time to change the practical aspects of the abortion legislation, particularly with regard to late abortions around weeks 21 to 22 of pregnancy. As a rule this involves about ten women each year who have been granted permission by the Council to have an abortion on serious medical grounds. However, there are also a few cases where abortion is allowed exclusively on social grounds.

The Legal Aid Council of the National Board of Health and Welfare expressed its views in a press release published on 15 May 2001:[7]

> There is to be no change in the stipulated time limits for abortion. There is no clear medical evidence available today that gives sufficiently secure grounds for a revision of the Council's present application of the abortion regulations. Abortion may be granted for special reasons up to and including but no later than the 22nd week of pregnancy. The Council emphasises in this press release that their decisions are taken solely on the basis of each individual case.

In cases where a woman has to be admitted to hospital in connection with an abortion and stays overnight, her data, including her personal identity number, are entered in the Inpatient Register of the National Board of Health and Welfare. All diagnoses and treatments received while under inpatient care are registered here, as has been the practice for several decades.

Some individuals consider that if all abortions that are performed before the end of week 18 of pregnancy are registered in the Inpatient Register, this is an offence against the Abortion Act. Others consider that this Inpatient Register is important because it is needed for the development of better methods and for keeping records of any harmful effects of different surgical procedures and treatments. During the approximately 40 years since the establishment of the Inpatient Register, the National Board of Health and Welfare has not noted a single case of misuse of its existing registered information. However, it has been suggested that an investigation should be initiated to determine whether or not the register could be regarded as a violation of women's privacy.

Selective abortion on the grounds of 'wrong' sex of the child

In recent years some opponents of the right to abortion have pointed out in the media that it is possible to abort female fetuses just because they are female – a form of 'gender-selective' abortion. The Swedish legislation says nothing about this, and no statistical data are available.

In a debate article in the Swedish newspaper *Dagens Nyheter*, published in July 1998, Professor M Bygdeman provided detailed information relating to this question.[8] He pointed out that there are three methods for ascertaining the gender of an unborn child:

● amniocentesis (i.e. taking a sample of the amniotic fluid)
● taking a sample from the placenta
● ultrasound scanning.

Amniotic fluid samples and placenta samples are normally only taken on medical grounds, and the procedures are not entirely free from the risk of complications. The parents cannot therefore demand such an investigation simply in order to find out the gender of their child. In practice the result of an analysis of such samples would not normally be available until after week 18 of pregnancy, by which time a special reason would be required for the woman to have an abortion – and of course a desire to know the gender of the child would not constitute a special reason.

Ultrasound scanning, in order to establish the gender of the child with certainty, would need to be performed so late in the pregnancy that again the results could not influence the decision as to whether or not to have an abortion. Thus the risk of performing an abortion in Sweden because the child is of the wrong gender is virtually non-existent. However, it is well known that selective abortion does occur in some countries, including India and China, where considerably fewer girls than boys are born.

Statistical information

World Health Organization statistics

According to statistics from the World Health Organization (WHO), approximately 20 million illegal abortions take place worldwide every year. In those countries where there is no legal right to free abortion, women have to pay large sums for operations that are carried out by laymen, with a risk of serious infections, and often with their lives at stake. It is estimated that at least 100 000 women worldwide die every year as a result of complications caused by illegal abortion.[9]

The situation in Sweden before the 1975 Abortion Act

In 1938, when the first Swedish legislation on abortion came into force, the number of legal abortions performed in Sweden was very small. However, the number of illegal abortions was estimated to be between 10 000 and 20 000 per year. In 1940, of those women who sought a legal abortion in Stockholm, but were refused this, 51% had an illegal abortion instead.[10]

During the 1940s the number of legal abortions increased, and by the early 1950s it had reached approximately 6000 per year. In the early 1960s, as mentioned before, thousands of Swedish women travelled to Poland. From the 1960s onwards, views on sexuality and premarital sex became more liberal, and at the same time there was a large increase in the number of abortions.

The period following the 1975 Abortion Act

Abortion care in Sweden is of a very high standard, and there are very few cases of complications. Approximately one in four pregnancies (25%) is terminated by abortion. Since the present Abortion Act came into force in 1975 the average number of abortions has been around 30 000 per year,[11] although in some years it has been up to 38 000. In 2004, the most recent year for which records are available, 34 454 abortions were performed in Sweden.

Today more than 90% (93.5% in February 2004) of all abortions are performed before the end of week 12 of pregnancy. Abortions performed after week 18 represent 0.7% of the total number.

From 1975 to 1985 the number of teenage abortions decreased. Since 1985, the figures have risen, fallen and risen again. The pill is the contraceptive most commonly used by younger women in Sweden, but its frequency of use has varied considerably over the past 25 years. Concern about side-effects has had a great impact on the use of the pill, which in turn has affected the number of abortions.

Compared with the figures for 1995, teenage abortions have now risen by approximately 50%, which means that each year approximately 25 in every 1000 girls undergo an abortion.[12–14] This increase is linked to the different reports on the association of the pill with thrombosis and breast cancer.

The significance of subsidising the cost of the pill for young women has also attracted attention during the last decade, and research has shown that it is directly related to the number of abortions. In a study[15] of young women it was found that subsidising the cost of oral contraceptive pills for teenagers reduced the number of legal abortions in that age group by 34% compared with the corresponding figures for the year before this subsidisation was introduced.

Reports of a further increase in the number of teenage abortions appeared in the media in September 2002, when it was stated that the number of teenage abortions had increased for the seventh year in succession. This was despite the fact that sales of the pill, condoms and the morning-after pill had risen during the same period. However, in 2003 and 2004 there was a downward trend compared with the previous year, and the number of teenage abortions decreased by nearly 4.5%.

In Sweden abortion rates vary widely according to geographical region, but the highest incidence has been noted on Gotland (a large island) and in Göteborg and Malmö (two metropolitan areas).

Abortion in other countries

Many women around the world live in countries where abortion is forbidden except in certain highly controlled cases. The laws and regulations vary considerably from one country to another. For example, the term 'risk to the woman's health' is interpreted in different ways. In many of these countries abortion is regarded as a criminal offence, and both the person who performs the abortion and the woman who has the abortion can be punished. The distribution of women worldwide according to the possibility of their having an abortion is approximately as follows.[16]

- About 25% live in countries where abortion is forbidden (or is possibly permitted in order to save the woman's life or, in some countries, following rape).

- About 10% live in countries where an abortion may be performed for medical reasons if the pregnancy is shown to constitute a serious threat to the woman's health.
- About 4% live in countries where abortion is allowed mainly to protect the woman's mental health.
- About 20% live in countries where abortion is permitted for socio-economic reasons.
- Just over 40% live in countries where they are entitled to free abortion (with or without restrictions).

On International Midwives Day, which falls on 5 May, a day devoted specifically to the subject of abortion was organised in Stockholm in the year 2003. Among other topics discussed was the possibility that women from other countries could have an abortion performed in Sweden. The opinion was expressed that an abortion cannot be regarded as being different from other forms of healthcare, and that it is therefore obvious that a woman should be permitted to have an abortion performed in a different European Union (EU) country from that in which she is resident, irrespective of her nationality.[17] At the conference it was also pointed out that there are certain criteria that give a non-Swedish woman the right to an abortion in Sweden.

In addition, it was stated that the most important point was that women must have the opportunity to have a *safe* abortion, regardless of whether it is legal or not. This would reduce abortion-related illnesses, suffering and deaths among women worldwide.[18]

The abortion process

According to Swedish law, the right to abortion in Sweden applies to women who are either Swedish citizens or resident in Sweden. The abortion must be performed by a fully qualified physician and should take place at a general hospital or other healthcare establishment that is approved by the National Board of Health and Welfare.

In their general directives,[6] the National Board of Health and Welfare state that the hospital should be easily accessible and that telephone lines should be open for sufficient hours to enable women to make an appointment for a medical examination. Women who are to undergo an abortion should be offered counselling before the procedure. As a rule, the father is also welcome to be present at the counselling.

After week 18 of pregnancy, a special case report must be prepared by a social welfare officer and sent to the National Board of Health and Welfare for evaluation and approval of the requested abortion.

Different types of abortion procedures

Early abortion

In cases of early abortion the woman may choose between a medical or a surgical method. A medical abortion must be performed before the end of week 9 of pregnancy. Otherwise, an early abortion is defined as an abortion performed before the end of week 12 of pregnancy. Irrespective of the method that the woman chooses, the procedure is normally performed at an outpatient clinic, which means a 4- to 8-hour stay at the hospital. Only in rare cases does the woman need to stay in overnight.

Medical abortion

The medical method that was developed at the Karolinska Hospital in Stockholm and has been available since the early 1990s can be applied up to the end of the ninth week of pregnancy, estimated from the first day of the last menstrual period. This method is considered to be particularly suitable for women who have given birth previously.

The woman needs to take a drug (mifepristone/RU-48 taken orally in tablet form) that will initiate the abortion process. This drug counteracts the effect of the hormone (progesterone) that protects the pregnancy.

The woman is then allowed home for two days, after which she returns to the hospital. She is then treated with the hormone prostaglandin (Cytotec or Cervagen, taken either orally in tablet form or as a vaginal suppository), which starts the uterine contractions. Pain relief is usually required. After a number of hours bleeding begins, and this is followed by a miscarriage. The woman generally remains under observation for 4 to 6 hours. Two to three weeks later she returns for a follow-up examination.

This so-called 'medical abortion' may be compared to a miscarriage with heavy bleeding, but there are seldom any side-effects (for example, infection is very rare). In 95–97% of cases the treatment results in a complete abortion. However, in rare cases curettage is required to remove remaining material from the womb.

Medical abortion has been accepted and registered by the EU since 1999–2000, and is used today in almost all of the EU countries except those that are directly opposed to abortion, such as Poland, Portugal and Ireland.

In Sweden, only doctors qualified in gynaecology are allowed to perform surgical abortions. This also applies to medical abortions, but in these cases the midwife has considerable joint responsibility. It is now being argued that midwives with adequate specialist training should be allowed to perform medical abortions.

As a medical abortion must be performed before the end of the ninth week of pregnancy, and the earlier it is performed the gentler the procedure, every effort should be made to treat the woman as early as possible once the decision has been made to proceed with abortion. The waiting time for a doctor's appointment is often at least 2 weeks, which can delay and in the worst-case scenario make it impossible for the woman to have this type of termination.

Surgical abortion

A surgical abortion may be performed up until the end of weeks 12–13 of pregnancy. Like medical abortion, it is usually performed in an outpatient clinic, which means that the woman does not need to remain in the clinic for more than half a day to a day.

At some hospitals, women who have not given birth previously are pre-treated with a laminaria tent. This is a cone of dried seaweed that is inserted vaginally into the cervix and during the following 4 hours absorbs water, expands and dilates the cervix.

Many women have found this method very painful, and therefore the hormone prostaglandin is now used instead for pre-treatment in many clinics. After this, a vacuum extractor is normally used. A tubular instrument is inserted into the uterus and connected to a vacuum tube, and the fetus is then removed by suction. The operation can be done under either local or general anaesthesia. It is performed by a gynaecologist and takes about 10 minutes, after which the woman remains under observation at the hospital for a few hours. Side-effects such as sterility are very unusual after a surgical abortion.

Late abortion

After the end of week 13 of pregnancy (defined as late abortion), the method of termination becomes more extensive and complicated, as there is some risk of damage to the cervix or uterus. Thus a late abortion involves a greater medical risk and is also a more painful experience for the woman, both physically and psychologically, as it is more like a minor delivery. In such cases the abortion takes place in two or three steps and the woman must be hospitalised as, for example, she may require pain relief. These late terminations represent only about 6% of all abortions in Sweden.

The first step

The woman is given preparatory hormonal treatment so that the cervix becomes softer and dilates when the fetus is to be expelled. This treatment takes between 12 and 36 hours and is generally not painful. During this time the woman may be at home or in hospital, depending on which method is used.

The second step

The uterus is stimulated to begin contractions. Usually prostaglandin is given orally or vaginally every 3–6 hours. After an average of 8–10 hours the fetus is expelled. It is unusual for the labour pains to last more than 24 hours. The contractions can be very painful, but different types of pain relief are usually very effective.

The third step

As a rule the placenta is expelled following the discharge of the fetus. If this has not occurred or the woman is bleeding, a third step is necessary. This consists of curettage, performed by the gynaecologist, to remove any parts of the placenta that remain in the uterus. In such cases the woman needs to stay in hospital overnight.

The people concerned with the abortion

The pregnant woman and her partner

The pregnant woman and her partner are the two people who are usually most deeply affected by the question of whether to have an abortion or to continue with the pregnancy. For many, the question of whether to have an abortion is not a simple one. This situation can involve both existential and ethical/moral conflicts.

Much has been written about the woman's thoughts, feelings and experiences in connection with termination of a pregnancy, whereas the men involved have not received the same attention. In recent years, however, some investigations have focused on the man's experiences when his partner has become pregnant (*see* Chapter 4). These studies have shown that the man is also faced with a number of problems, and in many cases experiences this as a time of crisis. The parents of the young couple can also experience feelings of conflict if they are told about the situation. The parents are often concerned about their child's education and economic welfare, and perhaps his or her immaturity in the face of possible parenthood.

However, the final decision as to whether or not to have the pregnancy terminated is in the hands of the woman, but she needs to express her feelings and consider any ambivalence she is experiencing about the decision. In cases where the woman and her partner succeed in connecting with each other in a common discussion about the different steps in the decision process, this may lead to a deepening of their relationship, or possibly to its dignified end.

The ethical dilemma of the medical care staff

The Abortion Act was initially introduced to help women seeking an abortion and their partners in the case of an unwanted pregnancy. However, many other individuals are also involved in the possible termination of a pregnancy, including relatives and close friends, the social welfare officer, doctors, nurses and other care personnel.

Often it will be a social worker who talks to the woman before she makes a decision about abortion, especially if it is a late abortion. The doctor performs the medical or surgical intervention, and the nurse and other care personnel are involved in the aftercare. These individuals have to consider first and foremost the ethical guidelines and the basic responsibility that they have for providing good care, promoting the patient's health and reducing her suffering. They also need to respect the patient's own evaluations. A woman who is about to undergo an abortion has the right to expect the same understanding and friendly attitude from the nursing staff whom she meets during her time in their care as other patients expect in care elsewhere.

Often an abortion involves a conflict of an existential as well as an ethical nature that can place both the nursing staff and the patient in a dilemma. To protect and save life and to sometimes assist at its very beginning are the ultimate goals of medical practice, and abortion is directly opposed to these goals.[19]

Lack of understanding of a woman who is about to have an abortion often has its grounds in ignorance about existential questions, different lifestyles and situations, and life circumstances, any of which may underlie the woman's need to have an abortion. Education and guidance of the caring staff are therefore of great importance, especially for those who feel ambivalent about their task.

In Sweden, if nurses or other members of the medical care staff find themselves in conflict with their own values and do not wish to be involved in an abortion procedure, support is available for them in a publication by the Swedish National Board of Health and Welfare entitled *General Advice on the Application of the Abortion Act*.[6] Here it is clearly stated that individuals who are opposed to the performing of abortions on ethical, religious or other grounds are excused from participation.

Disposal of the aborted fetus

Until 1990 all aborted fetuses were considered to be biological waste, and were handled as risk waste and placed in special waste bags that were sent for incineration. The need for new routines led to recommendations for more dignified disposal of the fetus, especially in cases of late abortions. According to the new recommendations,[20] fetuses from late abortions (spontaneous or induced) from the beginning of week 13 up to and including week 28 should be sent from the maternity clinic to the pathology department. Later the fetus is taken to a crematorium to be cremated, and the ashes are buried or spread anonymously. There is also the possibility of interment or of a burial ceremony if the woman or the couple so wish. In this case the mother and the fetus are no longer anonymous.

The right to abortion is here to stay!

Support for the woman's right to decide about her own body has grown progressively since the mid-twentieth century. With the passing of the Abortion Act in 1975, women with an unwanted pregnancy became free from disparaging treatment and arbitrary behaviour on the part of society. The right to free abortion gave these women the opportunity to carry on with their lives without fear of degradation.

Since the new Abortion Act was introduced, increasing efforts have been made to try to eliminate the need for abortion. For example, there have been programmes to follow up abortions, in an attempt to prevent recurring terminations,[21] and free advice on contraception is available. In 1988, Outpatient Clinics for Adolescents (OCAs) were established across Sweden. These centres aim to help young people to handle their sexuality and to prevent unwanted pregnancy and sexually transmitted diseases.

Today many young people feel confused and uncertain as a result of the sexualisation of our society. The media and the Internet are both channels whereby young people 'learn' about sex, not always in the best way. Many need help and support to resist the pressure from the media concerning so-called 'sexual freedom.' Everyone is also surely in agreement that the high number of abortions needs to be reduced, but most people are a long way, for example, from accepting the latest suggestion from the US administration (to be found on their website) – instead of recommending the use of condoms, they recommend abstinence.[22] For the majority of young people in developed countries this 'method' is a thing of the past.

However, there are representatives of some cultures and religions who view abstinence as a moral virtue – for example, Catholic priests, nuns and monks. Abstinence is also recommended for patients with certain illnesses, or those who have undergone a serious operation. Sportsmen and sportswomen also need to abstain from sex sometimes under special circumstances, and likewise those without a partner or those who are widows or widowers.

In developing countries, many individuals cannot afford to buy condoms. For them, abstinence may be the only way to prevent an unwanted pregnancy as well as infection with HIV/AIDS and other sexually transmitted diseases.

However, in developed countries where information and the means of prevention are available, a relationship between partners that includes sexuality together with responsibility, reciprocity, pleasure and joy should be recommended. If for some reason things go wrong, there is the possibility of an abortion. If a woman does not want to have a child at all, or does not want one just now, or not with the man she is with at the moment, she has an opportunity to make her own choice so that she can carry on with her life. *The right to abortion is here to stay!*

References

1   Swedish Academy. *Dictionary of the Swedish Language* (Swedish text). Stockholm: Norstedts Dictionary, 1998.
2   The Abortion Act governing termination of pregnancy. 1938: 318 (Swedish text).
3   The First Standing Committee on Legislation. 1946:30. Socio-medical abortion indication (Swedish text).
4   The First Standing Committee on Legislation. 1963:32. Abortion indication following the results of the thalidomide disaster (Swedish text).
5   Swedish Abortion Act. SFS 1974: 595 (came into force on 1 January 1975) (Swedish text).
6   National Board of Health and Welfare. *General Advice on the Application of the Abortion Act* (Swedish text). Stockholm: National Board of Health and Welfare, 1989.
7   National Board of Health and Welfare. *Statement by the Legal Aid Council for Legal Questions. No changes concerning time limitations for abortion* (Swedish text). Press release, 15 May 2001; www.sos.se/sos/nytt/press01/pmrr.html
8   Bygdeman M. Debate article (Swedish text). *Dagens Nyheter*, 4 July 1998.
9   Bergström S. Bluff about the population of the World. (Swedish text). *Dagens Nyheter*, 12 October 1999.
10 Hede M, Lekander N, Lodalen M & Yderberg N. *The Difficult Choice. A book about abortion* (Swedish text). Kristianstad: Bonniers, 1994.
11 Wilow K & Liber AB. *The Swedish Statute Manual* (Swedish text). Stockholm. 2000: 334.
12 Tydén T, Aneblom G, von Essen L, Häggström-Nordin E, Larsson M & Odlind V. Despite easily obtained emergency pills, the number of abortions does not decrease. A study of women's knowledge, attitudes and experience of the method (Swedish text). *Läkartidningen.* 2002; **47:** 4730–5.
13 Tydén T. Better sex education can reduce teenage abortions (Swedish text). *Aftonbladet Stockholm*, 18 March 2002.

14 National Board of Health and Welfare. *New Statistics from the Board's Epidemiological Centre: dramatic increase in teenage abortions* (Swedish text). Press release, 4 September 2002; www.sos.se (and search English text Abortions 2002)

15 Rahm V. Subsidised pill for teenagers – one year's trial in Gävle, Sweden (Swedish text). *Swed Med J.* 1991; **88:** 2296–7.

16 Odlind V. International views. In: A-L Pehrsson (ed.) *Experience and Personal Choices. A book about abortion* (Swedish text). Stockholm: Förlagshuset Gothia, 2000.

17 Rehn M. *Abortion [illegal], regulation of menstruation or abortion.* (Edited report from a seminar by Sundström K: Abortion in women's health care – a problem or a reproductive right) (Swedish text). The Swedish Midwives' Journal, *Jordemodern.* July–August 2003; **116:** 30.

18 Rehn M. *Abortion [illegal], regulation of menstruation or abortion.* (Edited report from a seminar by Zätterström C: The role of the midwife in safer abortion care – a global perspective) (Swedish text). The Swedish Midwives' Journal, *Jordemodern* July-August 2003; **116:** 30–1.

19 Bygdeman M. *Abortion in Sweden. Report No. 27* (Swedish text). Swedish Association for Obstetrics and Gynaecology, 1994.

20 National Board of Health and Welfare. *General Advice Regarding the Disposal of Aborted Fetuses* (Swedish text). Stockholm: National Board of Health and Welfare, 1990.

21 Mattsson I. *Development of Follow-Up Activity Within the NÖSO, North Eastern Swedish Care Sector. Report from the unit for care regeneration* (Swedish text). Danderyd, Stockholm. 1998.

22 Department of Health and Human Services. *President's Budget Increases Abstinence Program Funding: abstinence request in line with teen family planning money;* www.hhs.gov/news/press/2002pres/20020131a.html

Young women and abortion, their freedom and responsibility: their own narratives

Vivian Wahlberg

Introduction

This chapter deals first and foremost with the concept of abortion as a major and difficult question in the lives of many young people. The viewpoints of young people themselves, including their reflections on life, relationships and their future, are presented. They describe their experiences of the 'false freedom' of free sexuality, and many give their own examples of the difficult experience of facing the prospect of abortion, and how they felt in the aftermath. There are descriptions of sadness and disappointment about relationships that have gone wrong, but also many reports of feelings of relief and liberation after an abortion, and positive visions of the future.

Abortion: a major and difficult problem

Abortion is an important and difficult issue that affects the younger generation, among others. To a large extent it is young girls who have to face this problem when it arises, but boys are also involved (*see* Chapter 4).

The latest figures show that the number of teenage abortions in Sweden is continuing to increase. During the 7-year period from 1995 to 2002, the number of teenage abortions in Sweden rose by almost 50%. Despite the availability of the pill and other forms of contraception, the number of unwanted pregnancies therefore increased. Different investigations have shown that many young people have unprotected sexual intercourse, and that despite the availability of over-the-counter emergency contraception medication (the 'morning-after pill'), some women do not consider the consequences and they risk having an unwanted pregnancy. The morning-after pill may be either purchased from a pharmacy or obtained free of charge from Outpatient Clinics for Adolescents (OCAs) across Sweden.

In Sweden it can take up to 2 weeks to get an appointment at an abortion clinic or to see a gynaecologist. It can also take many weeks from the time of conception until an abortion can be performed. And what about the time period that follows the abortion? Where do the young woman and her boyfriend find help and support if they find themselves in a crisis? Unfortunately, some OCAs also have waiting lists. It is at times like these that a social network is very important, and that within their family and close circle of friends there are people in whom the young woman and man can confide.

Emotional instability is one of the many problems of adolescence, and this may be particularly evident in the case of an unplanned pregnancy. The process of deciding whether or not to have an abortion is often characterised by feelings of ambivalence and mood swings between anxiety and relief. Lack of support in such a situation may affect the psychosocial health of the individuals involved for a long time. This includes effects on their lifestyle, health habits, new relationships and future building of a family. However, an opportunity for them to discuss the problems as they arise can lead to insight and maturity in the future.

Thoughts about life, relationships and the future

Today most young people have a great need to discuss the meaning of life and existential questions. Unfortunately, there is far too little scope for such discussions, both at home and at school.[1] As a result, many young people find themselves isolated or even in crisis, and they become weighed down by feelings of meaninglessness or by existential problems, which can be brought to a head when they are faced with the situation of possible abortion. They have no real preparation for dealing with these problems, and the gulf between the world of young people and that of adults is often too wide to enable the two sides to reach each other and discuss deep and difficult questions.

My own contact with 18-year-old adolescents in ten upper secondary school classes in Stockholm in the early 1990s, in connection with a questionnaire-based study, provided clear evidence of this situation.[2] One of the purposes of the study was to gain a greater knowledge and understanding of young people's views about relationships and the question of what attitudes and possible taboos still contribute to the secrecy and concealment surrounding abortion. A further aim of the study was to compare the ways in which adolescent boys and girls experienced their roles in relation to sexuality and abortion. The questionnaire was to be answered personally by each of the students and returned within 20 minutes. Participation was voluntary, and no one was allowed to discuss the contents of the questionnaire or any personal associations until all of the questionnaires had been handed in. The completed questionnaires were placed in a large envelope, which was then sealed.

Lively discussions that could continue well beyond the time limit of the lesson began in all of the ten participating classes. In one class, discussion continued through the break and on through the following lesson, so that the teacher who was taking the following lesson was asked by the class if it could be postponed. One chemistry teacher was told directly '*We don't want to hear anything about chemical formulas just now – we are talking about **life**!*' Following some negotiation the teacher agreed, on condition that the chemistry lesson would be given after school hours. Discussions about relationships and abortion took place with honesty, depth and humour between mature, sensible people.

It was surprising how open and straightforward the students were in their discussions relating to everything from romance to family planning. They even raised difficult existential questions – of the type that they would sometimes contemplate late at night – such as what consequences can result from pure coincidences in life, what life's ultimate meaning really is, and how important crossroads in life could have a crucial effect not only on their own life but also on the life of their partner and perhaps that of a child.

With regard to abortion, serious ethical questions were debated, not least by the boys:

> Who has the right to my child? – If I have made a girl pregnant and she absolutely wants an abortion … I must have the right to 'save' this life and take care of it myself …

It is not unknown for men and adolescent boys to express a strong desire to take responsibility for a child whom they have fathered, and even to expect themselves to do so. However, Swedish law is very clear on this point. It is the woman alone who has the right to make decisions about her body and to make the final decision as to whether or not to allow a pregnancy to continue.

In this context I would like to mention a case in Italy that received a great deal of publicity in the early 1990s. A medical student had promised to accompany his girlfriend to the operating theatre and stand by her side to give her moral support during an abortion. Neither the girlfriend nor the doctors, who had given him permission to be present, had any idea of his secret intention – to try to prevent the abortion. Just as the operation began, he took a gun out of his pocket, raised his arm and fired three shots at the ceiling. He called out his innermost desire: *'I want to take care of this baby!'* There was panic among the staff in the operating theatre, the abortion had to be postponed and the young man received a heavy sentence.

The false freedom

In the study described above, the girls in the classroom often raised questions relating to what they referred to as their *'false freedom.'* There is much talk in society about the greater freedom of the young people of today compared with earlier generations, which involves a lifestyle in which it is expected that people will have sex with one another. However, the girls in the study were unanimous in their opinion that such 'freedom' is an illusion – a form of wishful thinking – as this kind of freedom often leads to demands and coercion:

> Just think about what happens at our student celebrations and other parties! Everyone expects to have sex with anyone around – with or without protection – no one cares! We have our freedom!

Many girls mentioned other problems:

> Boys expect to have oral and anal sex – something that we don't like to do 'directly'. And they want us to shave our genitals – it is all wrong somehow.

But it is the boys who make the rules, as long as they get what they want –
most of us girls don't even achieve an orgasm . . .

Such opinions are consistent with the observations of many midwives, namely
that young people often feel that they have let themselves down, and that their
innermost desire is to feel love first and not to feel compelled to have sex in the
way it is presented by the pornographic industry. Many young people never have
the chance to develop their own genuine sexual identity.

We also discussed in the different school classes whether and where there is a
safety net to protect young people against a sexuality that they reject, ways of
having sex that they do not desire, sexually transmitted diseases, and the use
of twisted representations of sexual behaviour, including brutality and vulgar
expressions. Who is there to give young people a contrasting picture to con-
vince them that many of them are going down the wrong road, and a dangerous
road at that?

Most parents in Sweden accept the fact that their adolescent offspring have
a sex life, and assume that they take responsibility for their own protection
against sexually transmitted diseases and unwanted pregnancies.[3] Thus there is a
positive attitude towards sexuality, and contraceptive advice is readily available
through the OCAs. Having a harmonious and trusting sexual relationship is probably more important for our well-being than many other elements in our lives.

Desire, attraction and love

In the eighteenth century the physician and natural scientist Carl von Linné
described desire, attraction and love as follows:[4]

> . . . in girls in puberty there appears a lustre in their eyes . . . The sight of
> or the physical nearness to the coveted person gives the man . . . the wish
> to have a more intimate contact . . . The person who is in love desires to
> have sexual intercourse with the loved one . . . There is an interplay between
> sexual desire and the growing closeness to a person of the opposite sex.
> The sexual drive certainly draws man and woman to each other.

The intimate interplay and growing closeness to each other that Linné spoke of in
the above quotation never had the chance to develop in most of the relationships
that were discussed in the student classes. Many students complained about the
casual associations that everyone expected of everyone else, which they
described as 'false freedom.' Many also stated that they blamed themselves for
just *'following the stream'* and for letting themselves down time and again.

An analysis of the above questionnaire revealed that many students wished
that a deeper and more intimate view of personal relationships could be
presented during sex education classes at school, rather than just addressing
biology and techniques. They regarded abortion as a very important problem to
be discussed, but expressed their feelings in different ways depending on their
gender and their personal family circumstances, culture and religious background. Their opinions were also strongly influenced by how much they had
understood of the sex education they had received at school.

Despite the obligatory teaching on sex and personal relationships in Sweden, there are clear deficiencies in knowledge relating to many important areas of contraception, such as 'safe periods', and also the risk of sterility. For example, over 50% of the students believed that there is a high risk of sterility following an abortion, although this is not the case.

The study showed quite clearly that within the area of sex and personal relationships, there is a need not only to answer questions about biological and contraceptive terms, but also to discuss questions about desire, attraction and love in more depth.

Many young people demand norms

We are living in a time when for many people the meaning of the word 'love' has become reduced to 'sex.' This has led to undermining of one of the highest human values. Love is not the same as sex, and the examples quoted above show that sex can sometimes be completely bereft of love. It is not love when one only uses the other person casually to satisfy one's desire and to gain pleasure, or even solely in order to be able to boast about one's 'conquests' to friends. It has been shown that many young people expect something quite different to this.

Real love involves reciprocity, consideration for the other person, and the courage to honestly test the way forward in order to build up something worthwhile and develop together. However, there is a real risk that many young people in early puberty will not have the strength to resist the demands and expectations placed upon them, and that they will instead just 'follow the stream.' Through the repeated contacts I have had with young people it has become evident that most of them are in fact seeking something quite different. They raise existential questions, they want to have deeper and more philosophical discussions about life, and they wish to have clearer norms and values for their way of life in order to create a meaningful future for themselves.

Abortion: when things go wrong

Some aspects of the abortion question will be discussed below, on the basis of both my own studies and my contact with young people (mostly young women from the upper secondary schools I have visited), and interviews and conversations held at a number of abortion clinics in different parts of Sweden. Some quotations from an interview-based study conducted by a midwife colleague, Ingrid Mattson from Stockholm, will also be cited. We analysed these responses and compiled them in an article,[5] and many of these quotations appear later in this chapter.

Sexual relationships and contraception

The majority of unwanted pregnancies are a result of failure to use contraceptives, or of their incorrect use. Studies have shown that around 70% of girls and women who have had an abortion admit that they did not use a contraceptive, or that they failed to use it correctly. Some girls stated that after a few drinks at a lively party they felt free to do what they liked: *'I simply don't care – it will be all right, the risk is not so great!'* or *'My feelings took over, all sense and reason sort of disappeared.'*

In some cases the girl had forgotten to take her pill some days earlier, or the condom had split and there followed a nervous time of waiting for the next menstrual period. Sometimes there can also be a nervous wait because the girl has experienced genital discomfort which suggests that she may have contracted a venereal disease, and she is anxious about what the test results will show. The incidence of several types of sexually transmitted disease has increased in Sweden, not least that of chlamydia, which without proper treatment can give rise to prolonged discomfort and may lead to sterility. Half of all cases of infertility are caused by chlamydia.[6]

Many young people reported that they had a positive attitude to the use of condoms, as they have both a contraceptive effect and help to prevent the spread of sexually transmitted diseases. The disadvantages mentioned by several people included the fact that they can be awkward and embarrassing to use in the act of lovemaking, and the possibility that they may burst or leak. Nevertheless, many girls favoured the use of condoms, which demonstrated to them that their partner was prepared to share the responsibility.

Many girls had used the pill but expressed some doubts about it in view of the risk of side-effects such as weight gain and occasionally feelings of nausea. As a result of the debate about the pill's side-effects, many girls were anxious about the risk of thrombosis, among other conditions:

> I am afraid to use the pill because of the risk of being ill, so we have used condoms except for just that one time when we didn't have one ...

Many girls said they felt that they are forced down a blind alley, and that there is no way that they can avoid having to take all the responsibility for contraception themselves. Some girls raised the issue of contraceptive pills for men, so that they could avoid having to take that type of medication themselves, but pointed out:

> ... I don't know if I could trust them to take them regularly. If you take the pill yourself then you have control over the situation and that feels safer.

Emergency contraceptive pills ('morning-after pills') have not really had the success in Sweden that was anticipated, but as information about them becomes more widely available, it is possible that in the future more girls will choose this alternative in order to avoid the need for an abortion later.

Reasons for having abortions

Those girls and women who have found themselves faced with the possibility of having an abortion are not a homogeneous group. Each has her own unique story that influences her thoughts and feelings about the decision. Several reasons may be given for deciding to proceed with an abortion in cases of unwanted pregnancy:

- it was a casual acquaintance
- the individuals involved are too young

- they have not completed their education
- they have nowhere to live, no employment, no income, etc.

In Sweden it is not true to say that abortion is used as an alternative to contraception. A woman who has once had an unwanted pregnancy is very careful not to put herself in the same situation again, although later in life there may be an occasion when it happens nevertheless. Among women of all ages, the statistics show that around a third of those who undergo an abortion have had one previously.

In Eastern Europe, especially Russia, views on abortion have always been extremely liberal. It is not unusual for women in those countries to have ten abortions or more in their lifetime. They have more than twice as many abortions as births, compared with around one abortion for every four births in Sweden.

In the above-mentioned interview study that was conducted in Stockholm in the late 1990s, and in my own investigations conducted among women seeking abortions, it was found that in most cases the woman felt that to have a child would be a hindrance because she was too young, had too little education and/or her social situation was too unstable. Another reason given was pressure from friends and relatives. As one young girl expressed it:

> I am having an abortion more for the sake of those around me than for my own sake . . . it felt as if there was no right decision . . . but only bad ones . . .

Another woman gave the following reason:

> I didn't want to hurt my partner. I didn't want him to know about it – also because this boy didn't want to have a child. Things felt really bad immediately after the abortion.

In a few cases the decision to have an abortion is made on medical grounds. For example, '*I discovered a pea-sized lump in my left breast, and I was told it was cancer.*'

The decision-making process

Almost all of the girls who had become unintentionally pregnant considered that it was important to be able to talk over the situation with their boyfriend several times before making the final decision. In those cases where the boyfriend had let the girl down, parents or close friends often offered helpful conversational support. However, the final decision with regard to abortion is always that of the woman alone.

Many women were ambivalent and remorseful about finding themselves in this situation:

> How could this happen and just that evening with just that boy? I will never be able to forgive myself for such a terrible mistake that can spoil my whole future. I feel upside down . . .

Many boys and men did stand by their partner and discuss the situation with her, but they rarely did so in as much depth as she would have liked. The girls and women often believed that their partner really wanted to be involved and to give consolation and support, but that it could be difficult for him:

> Sometimes he is very clumsy and confused – he doesn't carry a child inside him ... I felt very quickly in my whole body that something had happened. Most of all we both wanted to forget, but then reality caught up with us.

In some cases the women required a little more time to think things over, but only a few took up the offer of talking to a counsellor. A gynaecologist with more than 30 years' experience spoke warmly of the value of a conversation with a social welfare officer, something that had been obligatory in Sweden during the 1970s:[7]

> ... there is a need for supportive conversation during the most chaotic period, which most probably is before the decision is taken ... you feel tremendous anxiety as long as you still have two alternatives. It is also a way to begin the process of adapting, which everyone needs more or less ... today we do not actually have any form of supportive contact that is obligatory. It is almost a way of letting women down.

Unfortunately, many girls and women have the false impression that a dialogue would delay a decision or make it more difficult. In fact quite the opposite is often the case. A conversation with an understanding person can help the woman to see her situation from different perspectives. Such a conversation can also help to start the process of adapting to the idea of abortion before the intervention takes place, so that afterwards the woman can begin to put the experience behind her as something in her life that was unavoidable, and then move on.

Social network

Several of the girls and women involved in the studies spoke of their unstable family backgrounds – for example, *'I was brought up without a father ... I really want a stable family'* and *'I am a burnt-out child of divorced parents ... Today I am a little bit of a mother to my own mother.'*

The most important person in the woman's social network should be her partner, but there was wide variation in the women's narratives, which described attitudes ranging from deep compassion to forgetfulness, lack of interest and betrayal – for example, *'My boyfriend behaved as if nothing had happened ...'* or, as one girl stated:

> I was really disappointed in him. Partly I felt that it was his fault as he didn't use a condom and it was I that had to have all the trouble, and partly for the fact that he went away and then said that he didn't want our child. During the last week I wanted to get in touch with him, he could have changed his mind, but then he went abroad ...

Another young woman said with great disappointment *'I was so upset that my boyfriend gave priority to a ski trip just at the time of the abortion.'* Most girls described very clearly their need for closeness and contact when they were in this sensitive and vulnerable situation, and did not want to risk being abandoned at that time.

Many girls also described the need for contact with other adults, be they parents or some other adult person. One woman described the comfort and relief she had felt when one of her colleagues at work, who herself had had an abortion some months earlier, told her how well she had felt afterwards, and that she had taken a bicycle ride the day after the procedure.

Several of the interviews clearly showed that abortion is still taboo. One young woman said that she had told her father and her sister about her abortion, and that their first comment was *'But what shall we say to grandma?'* In other cases it seemed that the relatives wanted to turn a blind eye to the problem and avoid being too close to what was happening. In one case the girl's mother had promised to accompany her to the hospital, but changed her mind at the last moment:

> ... then I called my father, whom I had not planned to tell anything. He came along but didn't really know quite how to behave ... but at least he was there.

This girl went on to explain how much her father's support had meant to her, even if it was a little awkward under the circumstances. What mattered was that he had been at the hospital and had been by her side.

Alternatives to abortion

The option of having an abortion is not available to everyone, even in Sweden. For example, a woman may be unaware that she is pregnant, or have poor knowledge and little information about abortion, or she may have felt reluctant to make a quick decision and consequently the pregnancy is too far advanced for her to be permitted an abortion.

There are also examples of cases where, instead of having an abortion, the woman has chosen to continue the pregnancy. In some cases the child has been put up for adoption, with varying consequences for the woman and sometimes also for her partner. Some women find that they are constantly thinking about their child:

> I wonder whether the child is well and how it is coping with life. Does it have kind adoptive parents, and so on? I wish the very best for my child, but it is not possible to check this for myself ...

Many of these women also expressed a longing to meet their children when they had reached their eighteenth birthday, which in Sweden is the age at which the biological parents may have contact with their child.

In several cases where the couple had agreed that the pregnancy should be completed and that they should keep the child, the child had been a source of great happiness and much loved, and the couple's family and friends had been very supportive:

> We never believed that it would work so well ... old friends came with gifts and congratulated us and helped in every way, sometimes as babysitters when we wanted to go out by ourselves for an evening ...

Several young girls said that despite the epithet 'single mother', they led a good life, which was certainly not without difficulties, but:

> ... both my parents and my brothers and sisters help me, and it shows that they really love my baby. Often I have friends who come and join me when as a single parent I am very tied at home with my child ...

In those cases where the parent-to-be does not have a partner, friends or a supportive family, there are voluntary organisations in Sweden that work in different ways to support and help these women as well as couples who are uncertain when facing an abortion.

Alternative to Abortion in Sweden (AAS) is an organisation that was specifically set up to help women who are facing abortion, and it has local groups in many towns across Sweden. Information about its services can be obtained from antenatal clinics and libraries as well as via the Internet.[8] The staff include trained social workers, midwives and other individuals with relevant training. Girls and women are welcome to come along and discuss their situation once it has been established that they are pregnant and before they have decided whether or not to have an abortion. AAS gives advice and is able to put them in contact with support workers who can help those who wish to give birth to their child. Many good relationships have been forged with these 'advocates' for single mothers.

Different methods of abortion

Choosing a method

The different methods of abortion were described in Chapter 2. Young women who are about to make a decision as to whether to have an abortion do not always know what alternative methods are available. In some cases they may have been given incomplete information, and in many cases they may have been unable to take in the information provided, due to stress or other factors. Normally an unexpected pregnancy is such an overwhelming event that the woman needs time to consider her situation and a sensible person with whom to discuss it.

One woman, who felt quite lost, stated that '*I read the brochure at least ten times at home, and also talked to friends.*' Another said '*I had found out myself about the possibility of a medical abortion, but was never offered this alternative by anyone at the women's clinic.*'

One woman thought that she had made the right choice of abortion method (medical abortion), as did another who had previously undergone a surgical abortion: '*I definitely prefer a medical abortion to a surgical one, but in future I plan to avoid both!*' However, some women had a very different view, and one expressed her pain and uncertainty as follows:

> ... I wouldn't wish that my worst enemy should go through a medical abortion. The pain plus the uncertainty as to whether the abortion had really taken place was awful.

The above extracts demonstrate the differences in individual experiences of different types of procedure. For this reason alone it is worth going through the alternatives and having the opportunity to discuss them with a knowledgeable person, such as a competent and experienced social welfare officer or midwife, at an abortion clinic or a clinic for adolescents.

Time and availability

Normally an abortion should be performed as early as possible in the pregnancy in order to reduce the risk of complications and minimise both psychological and physical pain. However, many women reported experiencing difficulties when they tried to contact an abortion clinic by telephone, sometimes day after day. They stated that the worst thing was to hear a voice saying over and over again *'All the lines are engaged – please hold.'* In such cases it is clearly better to visit the abortion clinic in person in order to make an appointment as quickly as possible.

When facing the possibility of abortion it is important that the girl or woman (and their partner, if they have one) feels secure, can sense an atmosphere of calmness and has sufficient time to express their thoughts and feelings. Often they feel the need to describe the whole or part of their life situation in order to ensure that they will be treated in a positive manner and get the appropriate responses. Often a situation that involves the possibility of abortion is not a single isolated phenomenon but part of the pattern of the woman's life.

Experiences of an unwanted pregnancy

Reactions

Young people's reactions after being informed of an unplanned pregnancy are often overwhelming and difficult for them to handle. They require immediate help and support, and they need to be given clear and accurate information by someone who will listen to them and understand them. The direct quotations in this section illustrate the thoughts of many young people in this situation.

Dismay and anxiety

Most investigations have shown that young people often feel shock and dismay when they are informed about an unwanted pregnancy. Many are also surprised about what has happened. They know that in Sweden they have the right to free legal abortion, but they never believed that this would apply to them. Most of the young people studied approved of the fact that the Swedish law allows abortion, but many also had certain reservations:

> If you have a child then it should be planned, and the child should be born into a stable environment, which we don't have. It is good that it is possible to have an abortion, but it should not be misused – never again!

Many girls expressed anxiety about the future:

Imagine if I should have an abortion now and not be able to have children later on in life. It feels inside my body that the hormones have sort of prepared me to give birth to a child ... but that I am interrupting this and somehow fooling my body. Imagine if it doesn't work when I really want to have a child ...

Another girl said:

I have always thought that abortion is something dirty, something that I would never do. I don't think that I can be pregnant in the future ...

This kind of reaction was not unusual, but here a specific and very comforting answer can be given, namely that in Sweden it is very unusual for abortion to lead to sterility, as all procedures are carried out under completely sterile conditions.

A woman aged about 30 years told how she had been very doubtful whether she could ever be a mother. She had never had an abortion, but had now become pregnant in an unsuitable relationship. The anxiety that she had felt about perhaps not being able to have a child disappeared: *'the abortion was a confirmation that I can be pregnant.'*

Confusion, guilt and shame

Many young women have reported that receiving the information that they are pregnant evokes feelings of chaos, shock and confusion. Many also experience feelings of guilt and shame. They are ashamed of themselves for having been so careless with regard to such a decisively important matter – *'to give life and then to take it away,'* as one young girl expressed it. Another woman expressed her feelings of shame as follows:

... that I could not understand that sex without a condom leads to a child, it was so idiotic! I, who had read masses of information about this and listened to the sex education at school ... and then this happens – I feel ashamed!

A woman who had terminated her second pregnancy described her experience of the appointment with her doctor:

I sat before the doctor like the evil person who had already had an abortion earlier – so stupid to have put myself in that position again!

A young girl described how everyone lies there in the silence after their abortions:[9]

We suffer, we have pain, and we learn ... What have we done? Is it right? ... I lie here thinking about my crime, a crime that will soon disappear ... I never understood the risks I took, except when it was too late. I now understand. And I feel ashamed.

Some women also described other misgivings and recurring thoughts after the abortion, and how they remembered in detail certain events that would normally have passed unnoticed:

Sometimes when I pass by the children's sandpit in our neighbourhood and see other women, who are single mothers with children, I feel ashamed that I didn't believe that I could have managed as a single mother ...

Understanding and treatment

In recent decades there has been much improvement in our understanding of women who unintentionally become pregnant. There are harrowing descriptions from the years before the 1975 Swedish Abortion Act of how difficult this situation could be and how isolated and vulnerable young girls often felt. The Swedish minister and author Ma Oftedal has provided an example.[10] At an interview she was asked the question *'What have been the most important events in your life?'* The first thing she thought about was the abortion she had had when she was only 15 years old:

> ... it was unbelievably brutal. I had to arrange the appointments with the psychologist and the doctor myself. No one saw that there sat a terror-stricken child. No one cared. At home, from my family, no support could be expected. What had happened was a scandal and was to be kept quiet.

Even today, many girls are extremely anxious when faced with an abortion, and they have an inner dialogue with themselves about how everything will take place, and how the staff are doing their routine job day in, day out, and probably don't have the energy to show understanding and empathy. Many women say before their abortion *'it's just a matter of getting through this, of getting it over with.'*

There is clear evidence that in general the staff show great sympathy and consideration for the women who come to the clinic for an abortion. Very rarely does anyone feel insecure, criticised or discourteously treated. Overall we have recorded predominantly positive attitudes among girls and women with regard to their reception and treatment:

> [I was] very well treated at the abortion clinic, warm and understanding. Now, later, when I think about it I feel quite moved when I remember the great sympathy of the staff.

The abortion clinics receive many letters from patients. I have read a large number of such letters and reflected on their content as part of my research into young girls' experience of abortion. Many used phrases such as *'The doctor was so kind'* or *'the nurses were so understanding.'*

One girl sent a special greeting following her abortion, addressed *'To that lovely little lady at the reception desk.'* Apart from the name of the clinic, this was the only information she included in the address, and the letter did reach the intended recipient. In her letter the girl described how much it had meant to her to be well treated from the first moment, and stated that it was *'half the way to getting better – a friendly smile, a friendly question.'*

Many girls wrote about how their fear disappeared and they felt their human value restored after they had been met with such friendliness by the staff. They spoke of how it felt to be cared for, to be offered a cup of tea and a sandwich, and to be given an electric pillow to place on their tummy afterwards, which helped to relieve the pain. Many described the staff as 'angels', and many of the postcards received by the staff had angels as their motif. One example of handwritten text read *'Dear angels! What a wonderful friendly atmosphere you created.'* Another postcard had a picture of red roses and the following handwritten message:

> ... a red rose and a big hug to you all for your friendly voices, kindly smiles, your warm and comforting hands and your unending patience when I was in for my 'curettage.'

The girls' written messages described in different ways what the friendly approach of the staff had meant to them at such a difficult time. To be treated with respect and humanity, to have a hand to hold, helped them to get through that day and later helped them to put their abortion behind them and to move on.

Dreams and memories

The period around the time of an abortion is often characterised by dreams and daydreams in which thoughts and wishes about how life really should be are woven together:

> I should have completed my education, be a few years older and be in a relationship with another man – a man with whom I would really like to live and have children ...

One woman said that she had had many different dreams:

> I saw a lump of blood in a wastepaper basket the first night after my abortion, but lately I have had more pleasant dreams. One night I dreamt of a little girl who was learning the alphabet ...

One young girl expressed her desire to be pregnant again, as she had already begun to miss her baby. She spoke of a dream that gave her relief:

> After my abortion I dreamt one night that my little baby flew away on a wing – further and further out into the universe, and I felt a great sense of relief ... and thought that one day my baby will surely come back to me again.

Many women described their dreams and memories in terms of metaphors, parables, and elements that had special associations. One woman described her recurrent memories:

> ... feelings and experiences from my earlier abortion came back to me. I remember the odours and reactions – I have thought a lot about whether I should have looked at the actual fetus, but I never dared to ask at the time. There could have been something about this in the brochure!

After an abortion: rehabilitation

Relationships in the aftermath

The earlier in the pregnancy an abortion is performed, the less traumatic the experience is for the girl or woman. However, the decision to have an abortion is seldom simple and straightforward. Profound existential questions arise, and few people have learned how to handle such a problem. All of the woman's existing relationships are affected, but in particular her relationship with her partner. Some girls express negative feelings about continuing the relationship:

> ... sex, no, it will be some time before I allow him to be with me again. It feels so unfair that he avoided everything – while I had all the worry and the shame and the difficulties ... he failed me just when I needed help most.

It was especially difficult for those girls who had had a casual relationship that had not given them any real feelings of happiness or security. Some girls had agreed to sex, but only with reluctance as they found that it caused them pain or other forms of discomfort. One girl described her displeasure and disappointment as follows:

> ... it isn't worth the little I get out of sex, or the meaninglessness of it. Sometimes I have experienced pain from having intercourse – and then to become pregnant and then the boy runs off ... why does anyone actually agree to this sort of thing?

An older woman, feeling disappointed after her abortion, said:

> I wished for a peaceful and stable relationship, which I don't believe I will find with my present partner. It feels as if something between us has died.

However, there are also many accounts of the woman's partner being extremely supportive, and of a deepening and strengthening of the relationship between the partners as a result of the experience. Thus it appears that the support and love that a woman needs at this difficult time can be provided by the partner with whom she has a relationship.

The woman's relationships with her parents and siblings and with friends at college or at work can also change, and in some cases may even improve in this situation. Some of the women described being surprised by the unexpected understanding and help that they received:

> My parents and friends supported me in every way when my whole life was falling apart. They gave their time to allow me to express my thoughts, feelings and different motives/reasons for an abortion – it was so comforting when they just sat and held my hand ...

Several of the girls and women whose relationship with their partner had already ended had a girlfriend or an understanding mother sitting with them in the waiting room at the hospital. However, there were also cases where the parents dissociated themselves from their daughter's situation, tried to conceal the truth, or even lied by saying that their daughter was attending the hospital for some other complaint.

Many of the women who had faced the prospect of an abortion had found it helpful to be given the opportunity to talk to a social welfare officer both before and after the procedure, in order to obtain information about what takes place during an abortion, the anaesthetics that are used, issues of hygiene, and so on. One young girl who found herself completely alone when making her decision felt that it was comforting to be given support at this time:

> ... the boy, whom I met on holiday in Spain, knew nothing ... in my situation the social welfare officer became more of a friend. She didn't try to talk me out of having an abortion; she understood that I had no choice.

Change of surroundings

After the abortion many women felt that a change of environment, such as a trip away from their normal surroundings for a week or ten days, had a positive effect in that it helped them to gain a better perspective on their life situation. For example, if the woman and her partner took a short holiday together after the abortion had been performed, this allowed them to find peace and quiet in order to talk over what they had been through. One girl described how after her abortion she had gone to stay at her family's summer cottage for a week in order to be alone and undisturbed in a peaceful atmosphere. Another young woman described her experience as follows:

> ... but the best were the meadows where the grass grew high and the summer flowers bloomed. I am still fragile, but much stronger than before I went away.

One woman told of a long journey that offered privacy and peace: '*The trip to Greece was a comfort to the soul.*' Another found that '*it was rather good to get away, to stop play-acting, to get a little distance.*' Some women felt that they had gained new strength to enable them to start anew, to put the past behind them and possibly to be more attentive towards their friends, to explain to them what had happened and to warn them against ending up in the same situation.

However, not all women felt the need to go away. Individuals' reactions and needs varied. Some women said how relaxing it was just to be at home and to close the door and not be disturbed. Some women wept a lot during the first few days after their abortion, but after a while this eased, as if they had '*cried away the worst of the sadness and emptiness.*' Some women explained that they had a feeling like menstrual pain for the first few days after their abortion, and that they felt very tired.

One woman was surprised at her feelings, and remarked '*I don't understand how I was able to come home, sit down and have a cup of coffee right after the abortion.*' The feeling of relief now that the abortion was over, and in some cases the relief brought about by finally ending an unsatisfactory relationship, gave many women a sense of freedom and release.

Visions for the future

After having an abortion, many women daydream about the future and experience feelings of happiness as they realise that life goes on and offers them new possibilities. Perhaps a new vision of the future is born out of the feelings of hopelessness and despair. Yet at the same time they may often be reminded of what has happened: *'Just this Christmas my baby would have been one year old.'* They may also feel a sense of longing and hope that in the near future they will experience the joy of becoming a mother. A young woman described her thoughts as follows:

> I stood baking saffron buns for St Lucia day and thought to myself how much fun it would be if I could have the help of a small child. At that moment I felt a deeply personal relationship with my child and felt that it would have been a girl.

The desire to look to the future and leave the experience of abortion behind was described in different ways. For example:

> The world didn't end because I had an abortion ... I want to start anew. Of course I want a child one day – every girl does.

Often an abortion can lead to the personal development of the girl or woman as a result of the depth of her thoughts and the crisis that she has experienced, as well as the important and independent decision that she has been compelled to make. One young girl expressed this as follows:

> This is the first time in my life that I have stopped and thought about the life I live ... I had sort of coasted along before, and had been rather wimpish. At last I have been forced to think properly in order to make some important decisions and follow them through ...

What happens next?

New patterns of life

It is difficult to separate the two situations when one has firm opinions about something and then the impossible happens. There is an internal uproar due to the feeling of having failed oneself with regard to an opinion that one held earlier: *'I have always believed that abortion is wrong.'* However, as several women mentioned, when one finds oneself in this situation one sees things in a different light.

Many women had been faced with difficult questions and extremely important decisions involving different alternatives that might have negative consequences for three people – the woman herself, her partner and an innocent child. The women discussed the complexity of life – the large and small things, the fleeting and the lasting. Amid the stress and chaos of normal daily life, many less important things pass by unnoticed, but suddenly in this new situation everything becomes interwoven in a tangle of different threads that somehow have to be unravelled. For some women this can be a very difficult time. Many women were emphatic that this situation would never occur again. As one woman expressed it:

> I shall warn all my friends! Not one of them will need to accept meaningless sex and then go through all of this ...

Many women are extremely careful or wait for a long time after their abortion before having sex again, due to fear of becoming pregnant. As one of them said:

> I can have a wonderful relationship with my partner without intercourse – by cuddling and touching each other without directly having sex, so I don't need to risk becoming pregnant again.

The women's attitudes towards life, men and sexuality also changed after the abortion, not necessarily for the worse, but rather towards taking more responsibility for their life, their partner and their sexuality. As a result they experienced greater meaning in life and higher self-esteem: *'to sort of dare to take personal control of one's life and one's feelings.'*

The strength and courage to go on

Somewhere within us, beyond the stress, uncertainty and disappointment, there remains an unspoilt part that is the essence of the self – a core, a starting point for development and a source of hope.

The memory of having had an abortion often remains with both partners for the rest of their lives. Sometimes a discussion with friends about abortion or a television programme on this subject can cause a negative or hostile reaction. The memory of an abortion always remains in our minds, either hidden or near the surface, and from time to time will make itself felt. Therefore it is important to feel prepared at any time in the future to take up the subject, talk through the abortion again and 'clear away' any unnecessary troubling thoughts.

It is not unusual for a woman to say later in life that she has never told anyone about her abortion, and several such examples are described in Chapter 6. They clearly show the advantages of talking about the problem, because if one never has the courage to address the matter, the problem can escalate quite unnecessarily. What has taken place can never be erased, but women must learn to forgive themselves for the mistakes they once made, and then carry on with their lives free from any sense of guilt.

References

1 Leijonhielm M. Life and death in the school curriculum: the knowledge of life in two months (Swedish text). *Svenska Dagbladet*, 30 May 1955.
2 Bengtsson Agostino M & Wahlberg V. Adolescents' attitudes to abortion and family planning in Italy and Sweden. *Soc Sci Med*. 1991; **1**: 77–82.
3 Sundström K. Reproductive health from an individual and global perspective. In: P Ostlin, M Danielsson, F Diderichsen, A Härenstam & G Lindberg (eds) *Gender*

and Poor Health: an anthology on gender differences from a public health perspective (Swedish text). Lund: Studentlitteratur, 1996.

4 Ekenstam C. *The History of Ideas Related to the Human Body. Disciplining and character training in Sweden 1700–1950* (Swedish text). Gidlunds Bokförlag Hedemora, 1993.

5 Mattsson I & Wahlberg V. Follow-up conversation after an abortion. A qualitative interview study (Swedish text). *Tidsskr Jordemödre.* Norway. 1998; **7/8:** 22–5.

6 Byström C. *A Pamphlet on Abortion from RFSU Sweden* (Swedish text). Stockholm: Alloffset, 2000.

7 Wahlberg V. A phenomenological study on post-abortion syndrome in Sweden. Interviews with psychiatric doctors and Catholic priests. *Int Nurs Pers.* 2001; **1:** 105–11.

8 Alternative to Abortion in Sweden (AAS); www.Globecom.net/minna

9 Students at the Lycée Francais, Stockholm. We suffer, we have pain, we learn (Swedish text). *Svenska Dagbladet,* 10 October 1999.

10 Kihlman I. The collapse was the best thing that ever happened to me (Swedish text). *Må Bra,* 9 September 1996.

Chapter 4

Young men and unplanned pregnancy – risk behaviour and reactions: their own narratives

Lars I Holmberg and Vivian Wahlberg

Introduction

This chapter is based on a public health research study,[1,2] and it presents findings from a number of international investigations, and describes different theories about norms, attitudes and risk behaviour. These theories are discussed mainly in relation to boys and young men who are facing a situation that involves abortion, but in several respects they are also relevant to other young people. Narratives that describe the experiences of a group of Swedish boys and young men with regard to unplanned pregnancy are also presented, and the type of support required is discussed.

Earlier investigations

The teenage years and early adulthood are both stages of life when an experience such as termination of a pregnancy can have a profound impact on relationships and the mental health of the individuals involved. Many young men experience a situation that has been described as a life crisis, an integral aspect of the male human condition. The experience of being or having been a potential parent does of course differ from one individual to another, among women as well as men, and this experience can influence the ability to handle one's own future and family relationships.

In 1980 the Swedish Abortion Committee stated in its report that:

> Women do not willingly talk about their abortions, and men talk about them even less. But who is ready to take care of the man and his thoughts and feelings in connection with pregnancy and abortion? Where can he go to get help and support?

In its concluding remarks, the Abortion Committee stated:

> More research is needed regarding the feelings of the woman and the man and their reactions to abortion, as well as how abortion influences the relationship between them.[3]

There has been much research on the experiences and reactions of women with regard to abortion. However, very few studies have addressed the thoughts and problems of boys and young men who find themselves in a situation where their partner has become pregnant and the question of possible termination arises.

The findings of about 50 studies of the sexual knowledge and behaviour of teenage fathers, their attitudes towards marriage and childrearing, associated psychological issues and the consequences of fatherhood at this young age have been summarised in an article by Robinson.[4] One of these studies addressed the problem of abortion,[5] and the results indicated that most teenage boys wanted to be included in the decision-making process and to receive emotional and social support at that time. If they were not included in this way they felt confused and isolated. Teenagers who were already fathers had more liberal attitudes towards abortion than teenagers who were not fathers. They were more likely than non-fathers to believe that pregnant teenage girls should be given the option of having an abortion, and they also tended to want to accompany their girlfriend to the clinic and provide emotional support after the procedure.

The results of a national survey of adolescent boys in the USA in 1988 indicated that 13% of 15- to 19-year-olds approved of abortion in each of eight specific circumstances that were presented to them, while around 4% disapproved of abortion in every instance.[6] Those who had more liberal attitudes towards premarital sex and those who stated that they would be upset if they became a parent in the immediate future were particularly likely to approve of abortion. More than 60% of adolescent males did not consider it acceptable for a woman to have an abortion if her partner objected, indicating a possible gender conflict over the abortion issue. However, in nearly all countries in which free legal abortion is available, the decision as to whether or not to abort is the woman's prerogative. This is exemplified by a case in Oxford, England, where in 1987 the Court of Appeal turned down a male student's request for an injunction to stop his pregnant former girlfriend from having a planned abortion.[7]

A Swedish essay on 'The man's perspective on abortion', published in 1982, describes the results of an interview study of nine partners of women who had to choose between abortion and continuing the pregnancy.[8] It was found that the men's reactions were strongly related to those of the women. The author raises the question of whether in reality the man is not in the same conflict situation as the woman, but instead projects his own conflict on to her, in the knowledge that ultimately she will have to make the decision herself.

In a study conducted in 1978 in the USA, 35 adolescent males were interviewed in the waiting room of an abortion clinic.[9] Emotions and conflicts that were identified in most of the participants included striving for maturity and responsibility, concern about independence, and uncertainty about being able to provide for a child.

The results of a questionnaire that was distributed to 177 adolescents in Sweden and 223 adolescents in Italy in 1991 indicated that nearly all of these adolescents, both male and female, were concerned about abortion and its consequences.[10] However, this concern was expressed in different ways depending on their religious and cultural background as well as their education in sexual matters and personal relationships.

In a smaller study in 1983, more detailed interviews were conducted with four Swedish men who with their partners were facing the need to choose between abortion and continuation of pregnancy.[11] In the same study several social workers and physicians who were involved with abortion issues were interviewed. The limited study sample showed that:

- men tended to experience feelings of guilt when faced with the abortion
- men and women tended to influence each other when choosing between abortion and continuation of pregnancy
- men tended to need to work through their experiences and feelings when facing the possibility of abortion.

Norms, attitudes and planned behaviour

The norms and attitudes of young people influence their thoughts and reflections when facing an unplanned pregnancy. Some different theories with regard to these issues will be presented below.

Norms

Norms can be defined as rules which, among other things, affect our behaviour. Ajzen and Madden based their theory of planned behaviour[12] on the assumption that certain norms and desires to a large extent rule our behaviour and influence the choices that we make. They cite five different factors:

1 the expected consequences of a particular behaviour
2 evaluation of the expected consequences
3 ideas about other people's approval or disapproval of the behaviour
4 the strength of an individual's wish to do what other people want them to do
5 an individual's perception of their own ability, resources, opportunities and obstacles, i.e. their perceived behavioural control.

Attitudes

According to Jeffmar,[13] an attitude can be described as an integrated reaction to an object, a phenomenon or a person. The reaction is partly emotional, intellectual and/or cognitive, and partly behavioural. If there is agreement between what one feels, what one believes and what one in reality does, an attitude is formed. The duration of a particular attitude is partly dependent on whether the individual's actions in relation to his feelings and intellect are experienced as right and correct for himself and in relation to his environment.

Young men and risk-taking behaviour

Adolescence is an extremely important stage of development from a public health perspective, as the health-related habits that develop during these years have a major impact on the future health of an individual. Risk-taking behaviours include the use of tobacco, alcohol, illicit drugs or anabolic steroids, which constitute a potential threat to teenagers' health and possibly even their lives. Sexually transmitted diseases and unwanted pregnancies are two of the many possible consequences of a risk-taking lifestyle. The great financial burden imposed on society by such risk-taking behaviour has also been well documented.

Adolescence as a crossroads in psychosocial development

Adolescence is a stage of life during which young people face a number of crossroads and demands that influence their psychosocial development. As a result, they will hopefully be able to enter adulthood having developed independence, self-control, a capacity for intimacy and their own personal identity.

In early adolescence, around the age of 11–14 years, there is a need for separation from the parents, and increased identification with the young person's peer group aids this process. However, such identification may involve increased pressure to take risks.[14] The need for mastery leads to experimental behaviour, which often includes the testing of limits as well as risk taking.

The testing of adult habits is necessary for the mental development of young people, but it is important to distinguish between what is normal investigation and what can cause serious injuries and long-term negative consequences. Investigative behaviour in a safe and positive environment increases competence and self-confidence, but risk-taking behaviour jeopardises health and well-being.

We know that different types of risk-taking behaviour do not occur in isolation from each other but are interrelated. Boys and girls engage in different risk-taking behaviours, and their peers and family play an important role.

Social factors and risk behaviour

In the late 1990s a growing number of researchers focused their attention on the social characteristics and health-risk-related behaviour of male teenagers involved in pregnancies.[15–17] In 1993, the Massachusetts Youth Risk Behaviour Survey indicated that a history of a male adolescent being involved in an unwanted pregnancy clustered with other health-risk-related and problem behaviours to form a 'risk behaviour syndrome.'[18]

Biological development during puberty, which involves rapid hormonal, physiological and bodily changes, occurs in parallel with psychosocial development. Some researchers consider that biological maturity directly influences four psychosocial factors, namely intellectual potential, self-image, the perception of the environment and the individual's own evaluation.

Jessor[19] has identified five psychosocial fields which can be related to varying degrees of risk taking:

1 the individual's biological heredity
2 the social environment
3 the perception of the environment
4 the individual's own personality
5 other behaviour.

Protective factors

There are also protective factors within each psychosocial field.[20,21] These are not in opposition to the risk factors, but work independently and actively to promote positive behaviour and positive development. This can explain the common observation that many adolescents who appear to be at high risk do not succumb to risk-taking behaviour. They may also be less involved in such behaviour than their peers, or, if they are involved, they seem to abandon the behaviour more rapidly than their peers. The protective factors are considered to reduce the influence of risks involved in the teenagers' behaviour and development. For instance, they may operate in a cohesive family, have a social environment or neighbourhood with informal resources, have strict social controls and participate in organised leisure activities.

Common risk-taking behaviours in adolescence include spontaneous sexual activity without thought of or prevention of momentous consequences such as sexually transmitted diseases and/or unwanted pregnancies. A chaotic situation often arises when an unwanted pregnancy is confirmed, including the need to choose between abortion and continuation of the pregnancy.

Outpatient Clinics for Adolescents (OCAs) in Sweden

'Sveriges Ungdomsmottagningar', or Outpatient Clinics for Adolescents (OCAs), which were established in Sweden in 1988, stipulate that in order to become a member a clinic must demonstrate medical, psychological and social competence. This means that an approved clinic must have, as a minimum number of professionals on the staff in addition to midwives, a doctor (to demonstrate medical competence) and a psychologist and/or a social worker (to demonstrate psychological and social competence).

Almost all teenage pregnancies in Sweden are diagnosed at one of the OCAs (of which there are over 200), and most of them end in abortion. In 2004 the total number of induced abortions in Sweden among teenage girls was 6681, representing a rate of 24.4 per 1000 girls, compared with 1564 children born alive, corresponding to a rate of 5.7 per 1000 girls.

The incidence of teenage abortions varies geographically and is influenced by a tradition of early pregnancies and the level of unemployment. Over the years, factors such as the cost of contraceptives and concerns about the side-effects of the pill have also influenced the number of abortions.

A questionnaire study

In spring 1995 a questionnaire study was conducted at young people's clinics, which at that time consisted of 150 OCAs.[1] The purpose of the study was to obtain information about the opportunities available to teenage boys and young men in Sweden for obtaining advice and support during the process of decision making with regard to abortion. We also wanted to obtain information about how the staff perceived male attitudes and feelings with regard to abortion. The intention was to use this knowledge to develop models for giving advice and support in this difficult situation.

The questionnaire contained 15 questions covering the following main topics.

- Does the male partner usually accompany the girl when she visits the clinic, and what professional contact, if any, is available for him?

- Is the male partner routinely offered individual support?
- Examples of questions and problems concerning abortion raised by the male partner alone and by the couple.
- Common reasons for abortion.
- Opportunities for the male partner to influence the decision as to whether or not to terminate the pregnancy.
- Examples of concerns and common reactions expressed by the male partner.

Responses to the questionnaire were received from 121 of the 150 clinics. Nearly all of the clinics gave examples of questions and problems raised by the male partner. The results showed that most of the OCAs provided care of a good standard for the pregnant teenage girls, with opportunities for discussion and support by midwives, gynaecologists and/or social workers. In around 25% of cases the girl's male partner accompanied her to the clinic on the occasion when the result of the pregnancy test was disclosed (i.e. when it was confirmed that the girl was pregnant) or at the next visit. In most cases the couple was offered a visit to a midwife (95%) and/or a social worker (78%).

By contrast, only 16% of the clinics that responded to the questionnaire routinely offered individual support to the male partner. In those cases a visit to a social worker was the most frequent form of support, and the next most frequent alternative was a visit to a midwife.

As perceived by the staff of the clinics, the three commonest questions or problems raised by both members of the couple were:

1 concerns about physical complications, particularly sterility (mentioned by 49% of the clinics)
2 practical questions about how the abortion would be performed (47%)
3 concerns about secrecy and the divulging of information to parents, anxiety about the reactions of parents, and similar problems (44%).

Examples of common questions or problems raised by the male partner included concerns about the girl experiencing physical complications, the abortion procedure itself, a feeling of powerlessness, and difficulty in influencing the decision. Thoughts and anxiety about their own level of maturity and their age in relation to becoming a father were common.

Almost half of the clinics also reported that the consequences of abortion were either emotional or sexual in nature, and that a discussion of these with potential fathers, preferably by themselves, was required.

In cases where problems in the relationship were the reason for deciding to terminate the pregnancy, most clinics saw the male partner alone (47%), although in nearly a quarter of cases both partners came together (22%). A possible explanation is that it was possible to have a more in-depth discussion when the male partner was interviewed alone. Clearly an opportunity to express his feelings can strengthen the male partner's resources and facilitate an appropriate solution to the crisis, thereby reducing the likelihood of problems in the future.

Whether the pregnancy continued or a termination was chosen, many male partners experienced feelings of sorrow and disappointment. This may have been due to a sense of being excluded or powerless, or due to the fact that they disagreed with the decision. However, the majority of the clinics reported positive reactions when a pregnancy was allowed to continue, although the reason for this is not known. Perhaps more secure relationships or older potential fathers were more common in these cases.

The decision-making process

Nearly all investigations have shown that it is difficult to make a vitally important decision. Such decisions are preceded by the consideration of many alternatives – a process that leads to a final choice between different competing pathways. In order to understand the handling of problems by young people, especially young men, in the often chaotic situation that occurs when their partner becomes unintentionally pregnant, different theories about the decision process can be helpful.

Decision frame

Psychology and sociology researchers have described different ways of handling difficult choices.

A common method is to use a so-called *decision frame* with the purpose of giving the situation a structure and obtaining an idea of the consequences of different actions, results and possibilities.[22] The frame that a decision maker adopts is controlled partly by the formulation of the problem and partly by the decision maker's own norms, habits and personal characteristics.

What is right? What is wrong? What is dominating?

Another approach is to use the *dominance search theory,* which emphasises decision-making strategies that enable the decision maker to choose one alternative and adhere to it.[23] The person tries to build a dominance structure in favour of a preferred alternative. For this purpose they progress through four stages as they:

1 evaluate the alternatives
2 choose a promising alternative
3 test for dominance of that alternative over the others
4 if dominance is not found, the alternative can be made dominant by bolstering its advantages and de-emphasising its disadvantages.

These strategies may be realistic to different degrees and thus lead to good or less satisfactory decisions in terms of utility for the subject.

Major life decisions and free choice

Sloan[24] questions the existence of free choice in the making of life decisions, and argues that certain decisions have a special meaning for the individual who is making them. He calls these *major life decisions*. A major life decision is intimately

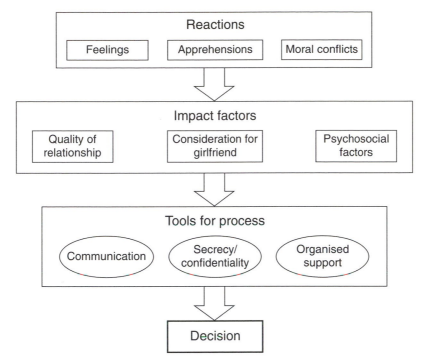

Figure 4.1   Model of the decision-making process with regard to abortion, for young men.

linked both to the question of identity and to authenticity. The decision maker asks himself if the decision to be made is an expression of his 'true self.' The term 'self-concept' is culturally dependent and therefore varies from one part of the world to another. We are often victims of self-deception. We are also very adept at rationalising certain behaviours whose expression has a deep meaning that we often do not understand, or of which we may even be completely unaware.

As mentioned above, risk-taking behaviour is part of the young person's normal development. When it results in an unintended pregnancy it leads to a situation where different solutions are considered, and individual norms and attitudes have a prominent role in the decision making with regard to abortion or continuation of the pregnancy.

Boys' and young men's experiences when facing an unplanned pregnancy

In 1999, in a Swedish study that was conducted using a qualitative method, namely the *grounded theory*,[2] 18 young men were interviewed at an OCA. They had recently been informed that their girlfriends had received a positive pregnancy test result. Ten of the young men were students, six were employed and two were unemployed. Twelve were living with both or one of their parents, three lived alone and three were living with their girlfriends. All of them were offered individual support by a male paediatrician at the OCA.

During the interview they expressed their negative feelings about the unintended pregnancy, which for the majority of them had come as a shock. The pregnancy gave rise to conflicting feelings, apprehension, and consideration of moral issues. After analysis of the interviews, a model for the decision-making process emerged that consisted of three concepts:

1 *reactions* (including feelings, apprehension and moral conflict)
2 *impact factors* (including the quality of the relationship, consideration for the girlfriend and psychosocial factors)
3 *tools for the process* (including communication, secrecy/confidentiality and organised support).

Reactions

Three factors, namely feelings, apprehension and moral conflict, became particularly evident during the interviews. Anxiety and concern for the girlfriend were also frequently mentioned by the participants. Lack of preparation and qualifications for fatherhood, economic factors and concern about confidentiality were cited as other important factors.

Feelings

The immediate reaction when the test showed that the girlfriend was pregnant differed between individuals, depending on their personality, age and other factors. Some young men had previously thought the possibility over, while others had not. The younger the individual, the less prepared he was for the idea of being a father. As a 16-year-old boy put it, *'It was a big shock, it really was.'* An 18-year-old boy said:

> Yes, it was somehow surprising, but perhaps not entirely ... I knew it could happen. But no, hardly to us. I was certainly a bit shocked.

However, positive feelings were also expressed: *'In some way I became happy because now I am sure that I am functioning and that she is functioning.'* Another young boy said *'My first reaction was – wow, I can ... I was somehow happy all at once.'*

The question of whether their partner would have an abortion or continue with the pregnancy caused feelings of obvious ambivalence in many adolescent boys:

> ... most of the time I have mainly been pondering ... I have not had so many feelings ... I have mostly been thinking of the two alternatives, there **are** of course two alternatives ... I have deliberated, turned over both of them in my mind ... I have also reflected on how life would be if we keep the child.

Too short a relationship and the young age of the girlfriend were mentioned as reasons for choosing an abortion. One participant in the study said:

> First of all she is too young ... and secondly, our relationship is too short ... I want to know her more in order to be a hundred per cent certain.

Apprehensions

In addition to having ambivalent feelings, many boys expressed concern about the possibility of their partner experiencing complications. This mainly related to fear of sterility as a result of abortion, but lack of confidence in the doctors' skills was also common. Furthermore, diffuse fears were expressed: '*Yes, I suppose I worry ... at the same time I don't ... but there is something.*'
Another young man said:

> It is something from me as well as from her that is taken away. It is like a piece of our love that is removed and that we have to rebuild.

Some boys expressed apprehension about their parents' reactions. A 16-year-old boy wanted his 15-year-old girlfriend to have an abortion, but she had decided to keep the child. The boy was very anxious about his own parents' reactions:

> I feel sorry for them, too, when I understand their strong feelings ... They are completely broken down ... I feel more sad as I know how they feel.

Moral conflicts

In Sweden it is very unusual to choose to continue a pregnancy for moral reasons instead of terminating it. However, the abortion issue gave rise to different opinions, ranging from '*I think it is OK. Some children shouldn't be born*' to serious doubts about abortion. The Swedish law on abortion, which permits termination of pregnancy up to certain dates, was generally accepted, but some participants had reservations about it.
One 19-year-old boy said:

> Yes, you cheat the body, you know that a child will develop but then you kill it – that is somehow wrong. In fact it was going to become a child – you cannot just ignore it.

Many men considered that from a legal point of view abortion was acceptable, but nevertheless had some reservations about it:

> If you are going to have a child, then you must have a stable home environment, and we don't have that now. It's good that abortion is available, but it should not be misused.

A 21-year-old man who had been strongly opposed to abortion, but had now accepted this solution to the problem of an unplanned pregnancy, said:

> Yes, then there is this disturbing element – if you are going to wonder a great deal, all your life probably, about what the child would have looked like and what it would have done today ... thoughts like that.

This man was disappointed by the fact that he and his girlfriend had insufficient support for them to be able to continue the pregnancy. He turned the matter over and over in his mind and said '*I think it is wrong that we cannot manage to keep it.*'

Impact factors: what influences the decision?

The next concept in the model is that of *impact factors* during the decision-making process, especially the following factors:

- the quality of the relationship
- concern for the partner
- psychosocial factors.

Quality of the relationship

The quality of the relationship between the young man and his partner appeared to have an important influence on the decision-making process. As mentioned earlier, too short a relationship and the young age of the girlfriend were cited as reasons for abortion. One participant said *'It's important to live together for some time and experience how that is before you have children.'*

An 18-year-old boy expressed the following feelings:

> I think that if you have talked to each other and are honest, then it wouldn't be any great problem ... I can influence her by telling her what I think and feel.

Nearly all of the young men mentioned that the decision-making process had led to more openness and closeness between the partners, and a stronger relationship. This is illustrated by the following extract:

> I think that we are more frank now ... we are a bit more close, I think ... maybe the relationship is stronger now ... the decision is so very important so you have to take care of each other, especially of her.

However, some men had experienced lack of honesty and considerable pressure in their relationship with their partner when there was a disagreement about the decision as to whether to have an abortion. A 25-year-old man stated that *'The whole time my girlfriend tried to persuade me that an abortion is murder.'*

Concern for the partner

A sense of guilt was described by some of the young men as being the initial emotion that they experienced when they were informed about their partner's positive pregnancy test result. Anxiety about and consideration for their partner were mentioned by many young men, including a 19-year-old:

> It isn't fair, when you are not intending to have a child ... she shouldn't have to suffer because of our mistake.

Other examples of concern for the partner included *'I will try to give her as much support as I can'* and *'I will give 110% support to my girlfriend.'*

Psychosocial factors

As was expected, the main reasons for choosing abortion were of a psychosocial nature. Typical reasons included inadequate financial resources, the need to complete ongoing education, and ambivalence about one's readiness for father-hood. As mentioned above, a 21-year-old man was disappointed that he and his girlfriend did not have sufficient support for them to be able to continue the pregnancy.

Recurrent themes mentioned by young men (*'too young'*, *'want to go out to see our friends, and find out things'*) indicated that they understood that they would be restricted if they had a child. This is summarised in the following extract from an interview with a 19-year-old:

> I think that you would destroy the best things in life ... maybe it would be enjoyable, but you shouldn't have a child for fun, it must grow up in a good environment ... and we cannot take the responsibility for a good environ-ment ... neither of us has a job – and our finances ... when you have a child you should have moved away from home ... established your own family ...

Tools for the decision-making process

The third concept in the model is that of *tools for the decision-making process*, and three factors in particular were mentioned, namely communication, confidenti-ality and organised support.

The girl has the unrestricted right to decide whether or not to terminate the pregnancy. Although this is a possible source of conflict, in our study none of the young men complained that they had no influence over the decision. Many of the participants mentioned that if they and their partner could talk to each other and be honest there would not be a major problem.

Communication

Opportunities for communication with the young man's partner, as well as with relatives and friends, are important aids to decision making about abortion. It is also important to consider the possibility of support from parents or, for instance, to obtain organised support from an OCA.

A 16-year-old boy stated:

> My mother was pregnant when she was only 14 years old, so she was aware of the feelings in that situation ... and she was not upset or angry either.

And an 18-year-old boy said:

> My mother is understanding and all right, so I think it could be an advantage to tell her. That would make it easier.

Nearly all of the boys mentioned that in-depth discussions with their partner during the decision-making process had led to greater closeness and strengthened the relationship. Despite the fact that ultimately the decision had to be that of the girl, many of the participants said that they felt they were able to influence the decision: *'I can influence her by telling her what I think and feel.'* However, there was also some uncertainty:

Two people are going to decide, but the girl has the right. In fact you can't tell her what to do ... You are in a way deserted ... I think it is somewhat strange anyway, that they decide ... she has it in her body, but the child will be mine as well.

Confidentiality

Two areas of confidentiality are involved in the decision-making process:

1 confidentiality within the clinic
2 the question of whether or not to inform friends and/or relatives.

There was a high degree of trust in the confidentiality of the clinic, although a 21-year-old man who had had negative experiences of social confidentiality said '*I am not worried, but I have to choose my words.*'

Apart from possibly telling a close friend or parent about the pregnancy, some participants felt that no one else needed to know. For example:

We feel that no one needs to know ... it's better to keep it as a secret. If you tell a friend, it may come out and that is unnecessary.

Organised support

This theme was not included in the question guide at the start of the study, but one of the men spontaneously mentioned when the interview was completed that '*It is very good to have the chance to come and talk to someone.*'

For some young men it is important to be able to talk to another man about their situation. This is illustrated by the following extract from an interview with a 23-year-old:

I felt ... outpatient clinic for adolescents ... women ... well! How can I explain – men and women think differently and do different things, don't they? Maybe men understand each other better, you don't have to reveal your feelings to be understood, you need to say only one thing, and that's enough. You don't have to go too deep, you can explain more simply and things like that ...

Decision making

The preliminary decision usually seemed to be made directly after a positive pregnancy test result had been obtained. In the case of some couples, where the partners had feelings of ambivalence, the decision was made after many discussions and a fairly long period of consideration.

What type of support is needed for boys and young men when their partner has become pregnant?

Most teenage pregnancies are unplanned, and relatively prompt decisions are required as to whether the pregnancy should be terminated or not. This decision is a female prerogative by law, but the male partner has a very important role in a number of respects.

The dilemma of the young adults

The experience of having to choose between abortion or continuing the pregnancy and becoming a father is different for each individual. The teenage years and early adulthood are sensitive periods of life when the experience of abortion can seriously affect intimate relationships and the mental health of the couple involved. It can even influence their ability to handle future family relationships in a positive manner. Many young men experience what is described as a 'life crisis', an important event in the male maturation process and of great significance for their future life circumstances.

Investigations in the USA have shown that most young men want to take part in the process of deciding between abortion or continuation of the pregnancy, and that they need emotional and social support in doing so. If such support is unavailable, they experience feelings of confusion and isolation. A similar situation exists in Sweden. In general, these young men take responsibility and want to take care of their girlfriends and participate in the decision-making process.

The experience of an abortion can be especially challenging at this critical stage of life when the young person's identity and moral framework are still being formed. If the partner's emerging feelings and reactions are not handled properly, this will influence their girlfriend during the decision-making process.

Support during the decision-making process

Interviews with boys and young men during the decision-making process have provided quite detailed information about what type of support they need, and what they consider to be important and valuable in this situation. Feelings of unreality, surprise, guilt and powerlessness are common reactions, but there are also feelings of happiness, and all of these need to be met with understanding and kindness.

In this situation the young man is often not yet fully independent, is neither qualified nor ready for fatherhood, has no financial stability and often has not yet completed his education. However, many couples reported that the unplanned pregnancy led to greater closeness and a deepening of their relationship. This often made it easier for them to reach agreement about the final decision.

For some young men it is difficult and sometimes even inappropriate to tell their family or friends about an unplanned pregnancy. In these circumstances the opportunity that an OCA provides for them to talk in confidence with experienced staff members is greatly valued. Often it is an advantage if this support is provided by a male member of staff.

It has been shown that there are marked differences with regard to health, health-related behaviour and risk-taking behaviour between young men who have been involved in a pregnancy and those who have not had that experience. Furthermore, there are corresponding differences between the following groups:

1 young men who have never had sexual intercourse
2 those who have had sexual intercourse
3 those who have been involved in a pregnancy as well.[25]

There is a clear tendency towards riskier lifestyles in the second group, and the most high-risk lifestyles are found among those young men who have also been involved in a pregnancy.

This indicates that OCAs need to offer general health-promoting information to young men when their partners become pregnant or have a sexually transmitted disease. Private, confidential sessions with school health services should also be made available in order to provide accurate information about health risks, and to identify and offer appropriate support to young men who are at risk. This is of particular importance in view of the fact that risk-taking behaviour is potentially changeable and preventable.

References

1 Holmberg LI & Wahlberg V. The staff's views regarding young men involved in decisions on abortion: preliminary information from a study of outpatient clinics for adolescents in Sweden. *Gynecol Obstet Invest.* 1999; **47:** 177–81.

2 Holmberg LI & Wahlberg V. The process of decision making on abortion: a grounded theory study of young men in Sweden. *J Adolesc Health.* 2000; **26:** 230–34.

3 *Family Planning and Abortion. Experiences of a new legislation. The 1980 Abortion Committee Report* (Swedish text). SOU The Swedish Government Official Reports, 1983:31.

4 Robinson BE. Teenage pregnancy from the father's perspective. *Am J Orthopsychiatry.* 1988; **58:** 446–51.

5 Redmond MA. Attitudes of adolescent males towards adolescent pregnancy and fatherhood. *Fam Relations.* 1985; **34:** 337–42.

6 Marsiglio W & Shehan CL. Adolescent males' abortion attitudes: data from a national survey. *Fam Plann Perspect.* 1993; **25:** 162–9.

7 Dyer C. Father fails in attempt to stop girlfriend's abortion. *BMJ.* 1987; **294:** 631–2.

8 Holm B. The man's perspective on abortion (Swedish text). Göteborg: Psychological Institute, Göteborg University, 1982.

9 Rothstein AA. Adolescent males, fatherhood and abortion. *J Youth Adolesc.* 1978; **7:** 203–14.

10 Bengtsson Agostino M & Wahlberg V. Adolescents' attitudes to abortion in samples from Italy and Sweden. *Soc Sci Med.* 1991; **1:** 77–82.

11 Björklund L & Rubenson-Emanuelsson B. *Before, During and After: the man in the abortion situation* (Swedish text). Göteborg: St Lukasstiftelsen, 1983.

12 Ajzen I & Madden TJ. Prediction of goal-directed behaviour: attitudes, intentions and perceived behavior control. *J Exp Soc Psychol.* 1986; **22:** 453–74.

13 Jeffmar C. *Social Psychology: interplay between human beings* (Swedish text). Lund: Studentlitteratur, 1987.

14 Lewis CE & Lewis MA. Peer pressure and risk-taking behaviors in children. *Am J Public Health.* 1984; **74:** 580–84.

15 Alster A, Lamb M & Tavaré J. Association between behavioral and school problems and fatherhood in a national sample of adolescent youths. *J Pediatr.* 1987; **6:** 932–6.

16 Fagot BI, Pears KC, Capaldi DM *et al.* Becoming an adolescent father: precursors and parenting. *Dev Psychol.* 1998; **34:** 1209–19.

17 Stouthamer-Loeber M & Wei E. The precursors of young fatherhood and its effect on delinquency of teenage males. *J Adolesc Health.* 1998; **22:** 56–65.

18 Springarn RW & DuRant RH. Male adolescents involved in pregnancy: associated health risk and problem behaviors. *Pediatrics.* 1996; **98:** 262–8.

19 Jessor R. Risk behavior in adolescence: a psychosocial framework for understanding and action. *J Adolesc Health.* 1991; **12:** 597–605.

20 Garmezy N. Stress-resistant children: the search for protective factors. In: JE Stevenson (ed.) *Recent Research in Developmental Psychopathology.* Oxford: Pergamon Press, 1985.

21 Rutter M. Psychosocial resilience and protective mechanisms. In: J Rolf, AS Masten, D Cicchetti *et al.* (eds) *Risk and Protective Factors in the Development of Psychopathology.* Cambridge: Cambridge University Press, 1990.

22 Tversky A & Kaneman D. The framing of decisions and the psychology of choice. In: G Wright (ed.) *Behavioral Decision Making.* New York: Plenum Press, 1985.

23 Montgomery H. The search for a dominance structure in decision making: examining the evidence. In: GA Klein, J Orasanu, R Calderwood & CE Zsambok (eds) *Decision Making in Action.* Norwood, NJ: Ablex Publishing Corporation, 1993.

24 Sloan TS. *Deciding. Self-deception in life choices.* New York: Methuen, 1986.

25 Holmberg L & Berg-Kelly K. Health, health-compromising behaviour, sexuality and involvement in pregnancy among 18-year-old Swedish males: a cross-sectional survey. *Acta Paediatr.* 2002; **91:** 838–43.

Chapter 5

Young people's attitudes to abortion in Sweden and Italy

Marianne Bengtsson Agostino

Introduction

Young people are obviously a target group for any intervention that is concerned with reproductive health, either with a preventive aim or for research purposes. In a study in which I was involved over a period of several years, the aim was to compare attitudes towards and knowledge about abortions in Italy and Sweden. The first target group consisted of upper secondary school pupils.[1]

That study, which was conducted in the early 1990s among young people in Italy and Sweden, was the main source of inspiration for this chapter. It is not the scientific results that are the main focus here, but rather the humanistic and cultural aspects of the study.

The following description is divided into sections under different subject headings, most of which were included in the study. However, the scientific classification employed in the original study has not been followed rigidly, and instead some parts of the results and discussion sections of the study report have been combined, commented upon and updated.

Earlier studies on young people, sexuality and abortion

International perspective

There is a great need for support and education aimed at prevention of the need for abortion among young people worldwide. Abortion is still a health problem, especially in countries where it is illegal or where neither information about nor access to contraceptives exists. Around 99% of the women who die after an abortion live in countries in the southern hemisphere.[2,3] In Sweden, where much preventive work has been carried out, the abortion rate is still high, with minor rises and falls, indicating that there is a continuing need for information.

The preventive work is often made difficult by the fact that measures relating to sexuality, contraceptives and abortion are linked to deep and complex aspects of life. Furthermore, abortion is associated with both sexuality and female physiology, some aspects of which have been seriously neglected and in some cultures are even taboo subjects.[4] In some African countries where the social status of young women is low and unprotected, an unplanned pregnancy results in a definitive move away from the family, a school education and an otherwise normal life.

It was not until the late 1960s that abortion was described as a health hazard by the World Health Organization (WHO), probably because up until then abortion had been largely illegal, which meant that the health aspects of the procedure had not been evident. Hundreds of thousands of women who have died or are dying as a result of complications after an abortion have not received any special attention.[3,5]

During a major international conference of the United Nations in 2002 in New York, the need for better education of adolescents about contraception was highlighted. The hope was expressed that before the year 2010, information about prevention of abortion and in particular HIV/AIDS would be reaching the majority of young people aged between 15 and 24 years worldwide.[6]

Education about sex and personal relationships

The number of women who become pregnant unintentionally decreases with increasing level of education, and with increasing information about and access to contraceptives. A good example of this is the reduction in teenage abortions that was achieved in Gotland, the largest island in Sweden, in the mid-1970s as a result of three years of intensive preventive work. In the project 'Living Together', representatives from many different groups of society were involved, and the aim was to reach as many teenagers as possible,[7] which had not always been a priority in international studies.[8] In a recent study in Naples, the authors pointed out that more education is needed in order to further reduce the abortion rate. It was found that 25% of the women who were interviewed after an abortion had not used any contraceptives.[9]

In recent years the incidence of sexually transmitted diseases has increased in many European countries, as reported both in scientific journals and in the media. Young people are particularly at risk, and these diseases are more common among them than in any other age group.[10] Many teenagers have sexual intercourse without any protection against either infections or pregnancy. In the university city of Uppsala, a research study showed that seven out of ten teenagers (70%) had had unprotected intercourse, and that girls were more likely to initiate the use of condoms than boys.[11] In a study of teenage girls in Barcelona, the proportion of girls who were on the pill had increased to nearly 45% by 2001.[12] A study of teenagers in the USA revealed that they clearly lacked the knowledge necessary to protect themselves from pregnancy and HIV/AIDS, and that they seldom used a condom and the pill at the same time.[13]

What then is the most effective way to communicate this important information to teenagers? In a study conducted in the UK, the attitudes of boys and girls to two different methods of providing information were compared. The young people either attended a guidance centre free of charge in order to obtain advice without the need to make an appointment, or were supplied with information via the Internet by giving them access to specially prepared home pages. The results of the study, which involved quite a small sample, showed that boys preferred the use of home pages on the Internet, whereas the girls preferred to attend a guidance centre without an appointment.[14]

Outpatient clinics for boys

It is important to investigate the preferences of boys and girls with regard to different forms of education. Often boys have been neglected with regard to sex education, probably partly because there has been a surplus of women in the professional groups that have been engaged in this activity. Many of these women are midwives or teachers, who tend to base their teaching on a predominantly female perspective.[3,15,16,17]

In Sweden, some interesting results have been obtained from research involving outpatient clinics for boys.[18,19] At a time when gender is much discussed, this is an important priority. It is essential to broaden and test preventive interventions and to take into consideration the similarities and differences between boys and girls with regard to their needs for information and education about sexual matters.

Another Swedish study, conducted among young men and women who had been in a situation that involved abortion, concluded that after the abortion the men's possible need for support was generally overlooked. The same study highlighted the needs of men and boys for support by the staff when experiencing a situation that involved abortion.[20] In a comparative study conducted in the early 1990s in Italy and Sweden, the lack of participation of the men in such situations was manifested in a number of ways. These young men were seldom present at the antenatal clinic, and the staff also seemed to overlook them during the routine outpatient treatment that was established for young people seeking an abortion.[1]

Is it possible to compare experiences from two countries as different as Italy and Sweden?

In the early 1990s, a doctoral dissertation on public health focused on a comparison of the abortion issue in Italy and Sweden.[3] During the planning phase of the project, the question of whether it is possible to compare two such different countries was raised – for example, when interpreting responses to questionnaires or considering the social aspects of the problems that arise.

A detailed description of the similarities and differences between these countries is beyond the scope of this chapter. However, one example that illustrates an interesting difference between Italy and Sweden is the change in the number of births during the last 30 to 40 years. Nowadays the stereotypical picture of the large Italian family is but a memory, and the large families that might be found in Naples in former times are more likely to be found in Sweden today than in Italy.

Compared with Italy, Sweden now has a higher rate of births per woman. In 2004, fewer babies were born in Italy and Spain than anywhere else in the world. With regard to the birth rate data, the lower figures in northern Italy are compensated for by the larger families in the south. In northern Italy the birth rate is less than 1, whereas in the south it is about 1.2. The decreasing population is a cause of great concern and is much debated among Italian social scientists. The population will be considerably reduced within a few decades if the current low birth rate continues.

Background information

Italy is the main seat of the Roman Catholic Church. From the Middle Ages onwards the history of the city of Rome has been strongly associated with that of the Catholic Church. The development of Italian society and politics has always more or less explicitly been influenced by the power, politics and resources of the Vatican. The most important stages of cultural and social development in Italy cannot be fully understood without taking into consideration the major influence of the Catholic Church on Italian history.

According to the Catholic Church, abortion is a crime. During my own research, I was often reminded of the vulnerable social position of women seeking abortion in Italy, not least with regard to their care after the abortion had taken place. In a small hospital outside Rome, where abortions were always performed on Saturdays, the women had to remain in hospital for one or two days. On Sundays, when the priest held Mass for all the other patients on the same ward, the door of the room of these 'lost' women was always kept closed.

Both the former Pope and the present one have always referred to the natural role of women as that of child-bearer and mother. This view hinders the development of a positive family policy in which men and women are regarded as free and equal individuals. The impact of the Catholic Church on prevention of unwanted pregnancies in much of the developing world could have been considerable if instead of prohibiting the use of condoms and other contraceptives it had encouraged people to protect themselves against unwanted pregnancy.

The increasing homogeneity of Europe

In Europe, the knowledge and experiences of young people are becoming increasingly homogeneous, which has both advantages and disadvantages. This international young people's culture applies especially to changes in fashion, music, art, etc. However, the differences between countries are still large, not least between countries such as Italy and Sweden, which have relatively little in common and very different backgrounds. After the Second World War, large sections of the population of Italy were poor and illiterate. It was not until the 1970s that major social reforms began, including the legal right to divorce, abortion, contraceptive education, public medical services and a new family law (which includes family relationship advice, benefits for children, additional services for families, other services to help separated families, etc.). All of this led to fundamental social changes. Earlier on, at the beginning of the twentieth century, Sweden also had a population that consisted mainly of poor farmers, but in many ways development there since the 1950s was more straightforward and faster than in Italy.

Information as a preventive measure

The Swedish Association for Sexuality Education (RFSU)

Since the late 1940s Sweden has had a national association for sex education (RFSU). It was initiated by Elise Ottesen Jensen, a prominent and courageous figure whose fascinating journey through the realm of Sweden was both real and symbolic. She was deeply committed to giving people alternatives to the ignorance about intimate relationships and sexuality that prevailed at that time. Prejudices were often associated with sexuality and could cause many problems and much unhappiness.[21]

Elise Ottesen Jensen had started her mission when her own sister in Norway, who became pregnant out of wedlock, was sent to an unfamiliar place in another country to give birth to her child, in order to avoid bringing shame on her family. At the end of the pregnancy Elise went to visit her sister, and was shocked to hear her strange ideas about the approaching delivery. Her sister had no idea how the baby would be born. This experience marked the beginning of Elise's lifelong commitment to promoting knowledge about the body, soul and sexuality among both women and men.

In Sweden the events leading up to the Abortion Act, which came into effect in January 1975, were more gradual than those which resulted in the abortion law in Italy in 1978. In Sweden the first law on abortion on medical grounds was passed in 1938. In the early 1960s this was revised to include abortion on social grounds.

Today, narratives from case records quoted in the book *Abortions Then and Now*[22] rouse feelings of indignation. The book briefly describes the fate of young women who experienced unwanted pregnancy in Sweden during the 1950s and 1960s, when abortion was still only allowed in exceptional cases, and many Swedish women travelled to other countries, such as Poland, in order to have an abortion.

The authors of the book quote the women's own narratives, and also give a glimpse of how their request for abortion was met by doctors and by society in general. Even a young mother with several children, all of whom had been placed in foster homes, was denied abortion by a gynaecologist, a psychiatrist and a welfare officer. The woman lived in an old-fashioned one-room flat with her husband, who was no longer capable of working.

The Association of Demographic Information in Italy

In Italy, up until 1972 it was illegal to provide information about different aspects of reproduction, and it was impossible to advise women on how to prevent an unwanted pregnancy. In the late 1960s, two far-sighted and courageous Italian doctors (one of whom was the physician De Marchis) established an organisation similar to the Swedish Association for Sexuality Education (RFSU). They gave it the strategic name Associazione Italiana Educazione Demografica (AIED), which literally means 'Italian Association for Demographic Information', as a more specific name that included the word 'sexuality', for example, would have met with opposition. This organisation consisted of a few dedicated individuals who worked on a voluntary basis.

When the encyclicae of the former Pope (Paul VI) was circulated in 1968, with the title *Human Life* (*Humanae Vitae*), the physician De Marchis published a small provocative booklet that included a collection of narratives about women living in deprived suburban areas of Rome, entitled *Unhuman Life*.[23] The book was mainly circulated in association with the AIED, and it described the arduous and difficult lives of young women for whom frequent pregnancies, childbirth and abortions were a constant feature of their existence. The book also contained information about the visiting activities of the AIED. Women who in the late 1960s were living in the poor suburban areas of Rome were contacted by AIED representatives, who tried to teach them about contraceptives. Sometimes the women were also helped to find individuals who could enable them to terminate an unwanted pregnancy. Information about contraceptives, including condoms and intrauterine devices (IUDs), was also distributed by the AIED. Often the women spoke of their difficulty in persuading their husbands to use a condom.

In Italy, sex education is still not a compulsory subject in school, whereas in Sweden it became compulsory in the mid-1950s. This does not mean that young Italian people do not receive any sex education at all, but such education is not obligatory and does not cover the whole country as it does in Sweden.

The Abortion Act in Italy

In Italy the Abortion Act, which made abortion legal, came into effect in 1978. This was the final round in a prolonged political debate. The government health minister at that time was a Catholic woman. As soon as she had signed the law, Catholic opposition groups began to collect signatures in favour of a referendum on abortion, which took place in 1980.

The Italian people voted to keep the law on 'free' abortion, thus transforming the situation in Italy overnight. Abortion had been a crime prior to the Abortion Act of 1978, and the need to make the change as clear as possible presumably explains why in Italy (at least in the medical services) the word 'abortion' was immediately replaced by the term 'voluntary termination of a pregnancy' (interruzione volontaria di gravidanza, IVG).

A study of young people in Sweden and Italy

In the study mentioned in the introduction to this chapter, young people were the target group. It was decided that the questionnaire should be distributed to pupils in the last grade of upper secondary school who would be a suitable age group for the study. Most of the pupils had reached the age of 18 years, and those who were younger had to obtain parental permission to participate in the study. It was also decided that the questionnaire should be distributed to pupils in the theoretical study programmes. In Sweden the natural science and social science programmes were chosen, whereas in Italy most of the participants were studying the classical humanistic programmes.

Another question that was discussed at the start of the study was whether each of the two countries should be represented by only one town. It was decided that in Italy, because of the major differences in history and social structure within the country, a group from the south of Italy should be included as well as the main group from Rome. In total there were 141 participants from Rome, 82 participants from the smaller town of Locri in Calabria in the south of Italy, and 177 participants from Stockholm.

Characteristics of the study

The aim of the study was to collect data in order to ascertain young people's views of the abortion question in general, and also their individual opinions about related aspects and problem areas. One of the characteristics of the study was its bicultural focus, which was mainly an advantage. The two countries' own languages were used, and in Italy the questions in the survey were constructed taking into consideration the special policies of Italian upper secondary schools. In total there were 24 questions, and they were presented in short simple sentences. Most of them were of the multiple-choice type, in which the pupil chose between fixed-response alternatives, while a smaller number were of the open-ended type, with 5–7 lines being provided for pupils to give descriptive answers in their own words.

Examples of topics covered by the multiple-choice questions include the following:

- sources of information about sexuality
- knowledge of contraceptives
- demographic questions (number of infants born, number of abortions per year)
- the partner's decision before an abortion
- feelings about having children in adulthood.

Examples of open-ended questions include the following.

- What is your definition of an abortion?
- What are the physical consequences of an abortion?
- What are the psychological consequences of an abortion?
- What are the different experiences of the woman and the man?

The most important open question was 'What is your definition of an abortion?' It was hoped that the simplicity of this question would encourage the pupils to answer as openly and freely as possible. At the same time, when answering this question the respondents could avoid mentioning personal experiences. None of the questions were formulated in a way that could be interpreted as being directed personally at the individual respondent.

Results of the study

Attitudes to abortion

The responses to the question 'What is your definition of an abortion?' highlighted important differences between the two countries. A comprehensive analysis of this question resulted in three response categories with regard to attitudes to abortion:

1 acceptance/positive attitude
2 refusal/negative attitude
3 technical/neutral attitude.

There were considerably more refusals/negative responses in Locri and Rome than in Stockholm. Furthermore, as expected, a positive correlation was found between the religious background of the pupils' families and a refusal/negative attitude.

The majority of the pupils in Stockholm considered that the consequences of abortion for both men (59%) and women (81%) were mainly of a psychological nature, whereas the pupils in Italy more often pointed out the social consequences of abortion. However, nearly all of the respondents considered that both women and men experienced anxiety or distress in connection with an abortion.

Different aspects of sexual education

The study yielded more interesting findings in the comparison between the two countries than had been expected. In the small town of Locri, friends were the main source of information about sex and personal relationships, whereas in Stockholm the main sources were the school and teachers. However, 20% of the pupils in both Rome and Stockholm and nearly 2% of those in Locri mentioned that members of the family, mainly the mother, were the most important source of information.

Attitudes of taboo and disapproval were still quite common in the south of Italy, where nearly all of the participating upper secondary school pupils (98%) expressed a wish to have more information about sex and personal relationships, and for sex education to be included in the school curriculum.

Similarities and differences in family patterns

The main differences that were found in the study concerned the pupils' family background and religious affiliation. The young people were questioned both about their own religious beliefs and about those of their families. The greatest differences were noted between the families. In the south of Italy, 85% of respondents stated that their families were Christian, compared with 71% in Rome and 16% in Stockholm. A similar distribution and response frequency were obtained for the question about the pupil's own religious beliefs. In Stockholm, 40% of respondents stated that their outlook on life was not influenced by Christianity or by any other religion.

There were small differences in the occupations of the fathers, whereas large differences were found in the occupations of the mothers. Whereas the mothers in the south of Italy were usually housewives, there were virtually no housewives among the mothers in Stockholm. However, this does not mean that the women in southern Italy were uneducated. Many women in that region have received an academic education, which for various reasons they do not utilise in a career. The reasons for this include unemployment, family structure and social organisation.

One factor that is often mentioned in the general debate in Sweden when comparing the standard of living in different European countries is the age of young people when they move away from home. In Swedish newspapers the term 'mollycoddling' or 'mother's boy' (in Italian, *i mammoni*) has been used to refer to Italian boys who even when around 30 years old are still living at home with their mother. In Italy, young people still live at home in adulthood. This is regarded as completely normal, and is perceived as advantageous and enriching, although some Italian parents do feel the financial burden.

In Italy there is no equivalent to the Swedish opportunity to borrow money during education (study loan), and it is more difficult to find suitable housing, especially in the large cities, due to the higher costs and lack of alternatives available.

The desire for children in adulthood

The great majority of young people expressed a wish to have children after they had reached adulthood. However, the results showed some differences, although these were very small and will need to be tested again with larger groups. In all of the groups, positive responses about the wish to have children in adulthood were more frequent among boys than among girls. In total, 16% of the Italian girls gave a negative response, most of these in Rome. None of the Swedish girls gave a negative response, but 12% said that they were unsure whether they wanted to have children when they were adults.

Women, men and abortion

One of the aims of the study was to identify possible similarities and differences between the attitudes of boys and girls to abortion and related problems. Some of the results were surprising.

The main differences between boys and girls concerned their own self-evaluated knowledge – for example, about prevention of pregnancy and about the menstrual cycle. More than 50% of the Swedish boys gave the wrong answer to the question that asked at which stage of the menstrual cycle there is the highest risk of becoming pregnant. The Italian boys were much more well informed about this and similar questions. Differences between the countries were only found when the boys' answers were compared. There were no major differences between the responses of the Swedish and Italian girls.

Both the girls and the boys in the Swedish group felt that the psychological consequences of abortion were most important for women (86%), but were also important for men (59%). Men were considered to have two sources of anxiety – on the one hand their own conflicting feelings about the abortion, and on the other their anxiety about their partner. In contrast, the Italian pupils reported that the social consequences of abortion were most important.

The greatest similarity between all three groups, among both boys and girls, related to the question of whether both partners have the right to decide whether to terminate a pregnancy, with 80–90% expressing the opinion that they do. More young people did not consider that both partners had this right in the Swedish group (21%) than in the other two groups. The differences between boys and girls with regard to this question were not particularly large, but might indicate a certain difference in attitudes, which could warrant further studies. There was also a similarity between the three groups with regard to their opinions about the psychological consequences of abortion.

Discussion

During the past 10 to 20 years there has been a continuing debate about legal abortions in both Italy and Sweden, as well as in the rest of the world. In Italy, Catholic groups at government level have presented their positions, challenging the present abortion law. In Sweden, abortions after week 18 of pregnancy are particularly controversial in view of the fact that increasingly premature babies are now surviving.

Teenage abortions are more common in Sweden than in Italy, where the majority of women who terminate a pregnancy are married women with two or more children. The Bush administration in the USA is strongly opposed to legal abortion, a situation which obstructs the preventive work formerly supported by foundations and contributions, which are no longer granted as before.

The Swedish study illustrates the complex factors surrounding abortion and the need for increased knowledge and greater awareness of the problems. The preventive work will never be finished. Every day new adolescents are seeking an opportunity to discuss and understand their bodies, their feelings, and the interrelationship with the opposite sex. The attainment of a more sensitive and problem-free approach to sexuality will not be easy.

Individuals need support to enable them to realise their needs and wishes. This support can be individually adapted, but could also be initiated in different ways – for example, as a research project. A questionnaire that includes important aspects of a topic which affect the majority of young people seems to encourage their participation, irrespective of differences in their background. It was obvious how engaged these young people could become when they were asked to comment on their thoughts, feelings and knowledge.

The comparison between two different countries added another dimension to the study, as did the comparison within Italy. All of the pupils had been informed about the geographical distribution of the study. The pupils in the classics programme of the upper secondary school in Locri in Calabria were particularly enthusiastic about the fact that pupils in Stockholm were also included. When the pupils had given their individual answers to the questionnaire and these had been collected, a group discussion always followed, in which all of the participants had an opportunity to ask questions or to comment on the questionnaire and the questions that it had raised.

Many questions in the study led to interesting thoughts and discussions. One such area was the adolescents' lack of knowledge about demographic data. Few of them were familiar with the birth rate in their home country, or with how many abortions were performed there each year. The participants were fairly well educated, and it may therefore be asked why this type of information is not included in the general education curriculum. Surely it is important to provide young people who are already in upper secondary school with fundamental information of this kind.

Throughout the study it was evident that the participants were unfamiliar with the concept of men participating in the decision about abortion. The idea that the whole abortion question only concerns the woman still seems to persist, perhaps unconsciously. The need for the man to be more clearly involved in the different phases of an abortion became more evident during the study. If a man is excluded from participating from the beginning, and he does not assume any responsibility, the idea that the woman has to face her abortion alone will be reinforced. Of course a man cannot make decisions about a woman's body and rights, but it does not seem helpful to exclude him at this difficult time, when his responsibility, knowledge and involvement are needed.

In women's groups that attach great importance to women's rights, abortion is seen as a matter of freedom for women, and the participation of the man in the decision has often been regarded as an encroachment. This idea needs to change, not to cause antagonism, but in order to allow further analysis of these attitudes.

If we exclude the man, the consequence may be that the abortion will become the woman's burden alone.

In sex education lessons at school, boys were also often absent. The main target group seems to have been the girls, without any reflection on the consequences of this policy. The teachers are nearly always women, and this means that the boys do not have the same opportunities for obtaining a good balance with regard to information, the opportunity to ask questions, and identification with an adult of the same sex.

Young people belong to the most important target group with regard to contraception. The preventive work that has been carried out in Sweden over many decades can serve as an important model.

However, natural scientific knowledge alone does not guarantee a more effective alternative. The ability to think and reflect is a unique characteristic of human beings, and it is our duty to promote this and to view it as an irreplaceable resource that can be neither created by any scientific technique, nor bought.

References

1   Bengtsson Agostino M & Wahlberg V. Adolescents' attitudes to abortion in samples from Italy and Sweden. *Soc Sci Med.* 1991; **33:** 77–82.

2   McLaurin KE, Hord CE & Wolf M. *Health Systems' Role in Abortion Care: the need for a pro-active approach.* Carrboro: International Projects Assistance Services, 1991.

3   Bengtsson Agostino M. *Cultural, social and individual aspects of abortion. A comparative study in Italy and Sweden.* Doctoral thesis, Nordic School of Public Health, Göteborg, 1992.

4   Bengtsson Agostino M. Taboos and physiology of abortion (Italian text). *Antropologia Culturale.* 1993; **7:** 25–37.

5   World Health Organization. *From Abortion to Contraception.* Copenhagen: World Health Organization, 1990.

6   Perrow F. *Sexual and Reproductive Rights in the World* (Italian text). Rome: AIDOS, 2003.

7   Nilsson A. *Experimental Work about Sex and Relationships in the Swedish Island of Gotland, 1973–1976* (Swedish text). Stockholm: National Board of Health and Welfare, 1980.

8   World Health Organization. *The World Health Report 1998. Life in the twenty-first century: a vision for all.* Geneva: World Health Organization, 1998.

9   Rotondi M, Labriola D, Ammaturo FP *et al.* Induced abortion and contraception: survey of 576 young women in Naples. *Clin Exp Obstet Gynecol.* 2000; **27:** 47–50.

10 De Toni T & Fontana I. Sexually transmitted infections. *Minerva Pediatr.* 2002; **54:** 539–45.

11 Darj E & Bondestam K. Teenagers' views on the use of condoms (Swedish text). *Swed Med J.* 2003; **100:** 3510–12.

12 Dominguez Bienvenido M. Which contraceptives do we use? Current trends. *Rev Enferm.* 2004; **27:** 60–62.

13 Ott MA, Adler NE, Millstein SG, Tschann JM & Ellen JM. The trade-off between hormonal contraceptives and condoms among adolescents. *Perspect Sex Reprod Health.* 2002; **34:** 6–14.

14 Hagley M, Pearson H & Carne C. Sexual health advice centre. *Int J Adolesc Med Health.* 2002; **14:** 125–30.

15 Centerwall E & Nilsson A. Intimacy in the AIDS era: sex education from a Swedish perspective. *Scand Rev.* 1988; **76:** 1.

16 Holmgren K. Increasing abortion rate in Sweden. Time for sex speciality? (Swedish text). *Nord Med.* 1990; **105:** 46–8.

17 Gottlieb C, Christiansen I, Von Segebaden C & Wiksten-Alströmer M. Successful attempt with outpatients clinics for boys (Swedish text). *Swed Med J.* 1998; **95:** 3418–19.

18 Forsberg M. *Abortion at Outpatient Clinics for Adolescents. A follow-up* (Swedish text). Stockholm: National Institute of Public Health, 1999.

19 Kero A, Lalos A, Högberg U & Jacobsson L. The male partner involved in legal abortion. *Hum Reprod.* 1999; **14:** 2669–75.

20 Holmberg LI & Wahlberg V. The staff's view regarding young men involved in decisions on abortion: preliminary information from a study of outpatient clinics for adolescents in Sweden. *Gynecol Obstet Invest.* 1999; **47:** 177–81.

21 Ottesen Jensen E. *The Life Wrote* (Swedish text). Stockholm: Ordfront, 1986.

22 Davidson B & Forsling C. *Abortions Then and Now* (Swedish text). Stockholm: Bokförlaget Röda Rummet, 1982.

23 De Marchis G. *Inhumanae Vitae* (Italian text). Rome: AIED, 1969.

Chapter 6

Women's memories after abortion, summarised from therapy work, pastoral counselling and/or confessions

Vivian Wahlberg

Introduction

Abortion may be the world's oldest method of fertility control. Both planned and unplanned pregnancies and the desire to control fertility are human concerns of high priority and are usually regulated, particularly in the Western world. Compared with women in the rest of the world, women in Sweden and most other Western European countries are in a considerably better situation because of legislation which gives them the right to a free and safe abortion without the need for specific grounds (which means that the woman is able to decide herself whether to have an abortion), and the fact that abortion can be performed within the official hospital system.[1] However, the information and counselling services on abortion are still poor in many countries, both for women and particularly for men.[2,3] There is a need for both psychological counselling and general objective information about the abortion.[4] As was mentioned in Chapter 2, a new Abortion Act came into force in Sweden in 1975.[5] This was the result of the gradual liberalisation of abortion, which had started in 1938 with the legalisation of abortion on therapeutic grounds.

Although most women seem to experience initial feelings of release and only short-term psychological problems after abortion,[6] some experience prolonged feelings of guilt, regret, and sensitivity to comments about abortion. These women need more adequate counselling and support than are provided at the moment.[7,8]

An interview study with psychiatrists and Catholic priests

Study aims

The purpose of this study was to gain a greater knowledge of women's feelings, thoughts, needs and possible prolonged mental and/or spiritual problems after an abortion (sometimes up to 10–30 years afterwards). The main question was how this could be reflected by and summarised from the experiences of psychiatrists and Catholic priests during therapy work, pastoral counselling and/or confessions.

The study was granted ethical approval by the ethical committee at the Karolinska Institute, Stockholm. Permission to conduct and tape-record the interviews was then obtained from each psychiatrist and Catholic priest, all of whom were assured that any information which they provided would be treated with respect, and that the identity of individuals would not be disclosed.

Method

To be able to fully describe the serious and sometimes long-lasting problems that some women experienced after abortion, a qualitative method had to be used. A phenomenological approach was chosen.

Phenomenology is a philosophy as well as a research method. The word 'phenomenon' is derived from the Greek verb *'phainomenon'*, which means 'to show or appear.' In 1965, the philosopher Edmund Husserl[9] challenged individuals to 'go back to the things themselves' and see the everyday world as it really appears – varied and complex. The phenomenological method offers a new way to interpret the nature of consciousness of an individual's involvement in the world.[10] The purpose of phenomenological research is to describe experiences as they are lived. It is an attempt to understand the phenomenon – in this study, abortion – from the perspective of the individuals who are involved in it – here described in summarised experiences from therapy, pastoral counselling and/or confessions.

The method seeks to uncover the meaning of humanly experienced problems by analysing the individual's description. The analysis of data, by abstracting the words of interviewees, reveals the essence of the experience, which responds to the research questions.[11,12] Phenomenology involves four basic steps: *Bracketing, Intuition, Analysing, and Describing.*[13]

Study design

As problems related to abortion must be treated in absolute confidence, the geographical distribution of the study extended from the very south to the very north of Sweden, and included large cities as well as more rural regions. The study results describe seven psychiatrists' and 11 Catholic priests' summarised experiences from therapy, pastoral counselling and/or confessions involving women from both urban and rural areas. The interviews took place in the office of the interviewee or in a few cases in a borrowed office, and they lasted for 45–60 minutes. Four of the seven psychiatrists were female, and all of the 11 Catholic priests were male.

The psychiatrists and Catholic priests were all encouraged to describe their summarised experiences of and reflections on their contact with women who had had abortion-related problems. Such contact had taken place during the 10–40 years of these professionals' working lives.

They were asked to focus on four areas in particular:

1 their own summarised experiences (from therapy work or confessions) of working with women who had had an abortion
2 the characteristics of these women's narratives with regard to their thoughts and feelings after an abortion
3 the needs of these women for support, counselling and/or therapy
4 the needs of these women for more information about abortion.

Data analysis

The interview data were transcribed and analysed line by line according to the phenomenological approach. Each interview was first read through in order to obtain an overview. The descriptions were then read again and the essential meaning units were underlined. Next the meanings were organised into different themes by relating them both to each other and to the other content of the interviews. After reading through once again and reflecting on the emerging themes, the descriptions of the interviewed individuals were abstracted into a more concept-defined vocabulary. Finally, the essential structure of the phenomenon of abortion was formulated.

Results of the study

The interviews were conducted in 1996 and 1997. The summarised experiences and memories described by women who had experienced problems with abortion, which were revealed in therapy, pastoral counselling and/or confessions, were analysed and gave the following results.

The meaning units were grouped into five different themes:

1 guilt and shame
2 effects of family influences
3 effects of social influences
4 memories and sadness
5 insight/maturity after pastoral counselling and/or confession.

The themes do not have clear boundaries, and there is some overlap. Each of the themes had two or three sub-themes, which are illustrated below by extracts from the interviews. The letters in parentheses after each extract indicate

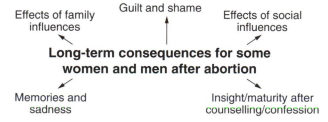

Figure 6.1 Meaning units grouped into five different themes, with the essential structure of the phenomenon summarised in the centre.

whether it is derived from an interview with a psychiatrist (dr) or a Catholic priest (cp). Finally, the essential structure of the experience of abortion could be summarised as the long-term consequences of abortion for some women and men (*see* Figure 6.1).

Guilt and shame

Guilt and shame seemed to be experienced by many women after an abortion, and several women appeared to have difficulty in conveying their experiences to the psychiatrist or priest.

Descriptions in metaphors

A woman spoke about a particular trauma that had occurred 12–15 years earlier in her life. She went backwards and forwards, using different metaphors for the trauma and how it negatively influenced her life. As soon as she mentioned the word 'abortion', it was like peeling an onion, to open up and remove layer after layer of repressed sadness and despair.

(dr)

Taboo, guilt and shame

I think that many events like abortion remain untouched for years or even decades ... it isn't easy to go to a priest with such a taboo problem even in the society of today ... Some women feel that they have deprived a human being of life – some feel like murderers, but there is no sin that will not be forgiven by God.

(cp)

No shame, but not ethically defensible

In the early 1960s many young couples decided to have an abortion as a matter of course – they just went through with it, and for many it seemed that there was no agony of conscience ... More recently the social climate has become more open to ethical–moral questions.

(cp)

Effect of family influence

Both psychiatrists and priests mentioned the influences of the environment and the family, especially pressure from the woman's husband to choose an abortion.

Pressure from the family

In some religions and cultures it is very important for the father that his family includes at least one boy ... thus there are abortions because a child is of the wrong gender – the negative side of our medical–technological progress!

(dr)

One husband said:

> I have had enough, I cannot bear screaming from one more baby ... You have to choose between me and the child!
>
> (cp)

In one case a young woman was forced to have an abortion by her own mother, who was also a good Catholic, but who did not want to have a 'false' grandchild.

(cp)

Freedom – disappointment – deceit/guilt

> ... it is almost a stereotype what the men can say to their women: 'Do what you want', which is one of the worst answers to get when she is in need of support ... it is an escape from his responsibility. He thinks he is being generous, but this is typical idealising of his own reaction, which in fact amounts to deceit or guile ... this is the exact opposite of love. Hate is not the opposite of love. Hate always has an active or positive core. It is a relationship, albeit a changed and destructive relationship – but it says something. However, deceit or guile is 'a nothing', and that is the worst!
>
> (cp)

Effects of social influences

Since the abortion law came into effect in 1975 it has been much easier for most women in Sweden to have an abortion. However, at the same time there is less control over the process, which has made it more difficult for individuals who are in need of more counselling and support, or who need more time in which to reflect before deciding whether to have an abortion.

Social support

> In Swedish society we have 'youth clinics' and we have 'clinics for abortion counselling' ... there is a need for help during the most difficult time, which is probably before the decision is made ... there is greater anxiety then because you still have two alternatives.
>
> (dr)

> Previously it was compulsory to have a counselling meeting before an abortion. In the 1980s when I was in charge of many abortion procedures, I felt that those women found it very helpful during quite a difficult and time-consuming decision-making process to be given time to discuss the problem and to reflect on it, and thus in some respects to work through the problem. For many women there is still a need for this compulsory counselling meeting.
>
> (dr)

Alternatives to abortion

I have a woman in therapy who is nearly 50 years old. Her mother wanted to have an abortion 50 years ago, but for some reason was unable to do so. This has had enormous consequences for her daughter ... she often heard that she was the unwanted child, and that she should never have been born. And she still feels unnecessary, unwanted, ugly and miserable.

(dr)

Sometimes adoption is mentioned as an alternative to abortion, but I met a woman who suffered a lot. She knew where her child lived, and she very often waited outside the day care centre to get a glimpse of her son. Her whole life is dominated by a feeling of great loss and longing for the day when the boy will be 18 years old, when she will have a chance to meet him as his biological mother.

(cp)

Provision of factual information and support

Of course, factual and preventive information is important both early in life from their families and at school while they are growing up ... Also later in life, if [a woman has had] an abortion ... to help her to understand that she is not alone. Information with different perspectives could help her to work through the situation and reduce her feelings of guilt.

(dr)

I believe that we must meet these women with great understanding and love and not put any more guilt and burden on their shoulders ... never condemn them! Try instead to give them their dignity back!

(cp)

Memories and sadness

Both psychiatrists and priests often spoke about long-lasting problems, and how these affected the women, and sometimes also the men, years or even decades after an abortion.

Reminiscence: grief and loss

... especially I remember one of them, a man who for many years came back again and again to discuss the problem. Despite the forgiveness he had received, when he met his brother's children he always thought of 'his own baby' who could have been a source of great joy today.

(cp)

One woman said, 12 years after her abortion, 'I have not only damaged and killed a baby, but I have also damaged my own life.'

(cp)

Relationship with husband and children, and sexual life

On special occasions they are reminded of the abortion ... one said 'For Christmas and other holidays there should have been one more in my family. The guilt and sadness after my abortion have taken away the real happiness with my other children.'

(cp)

A woman said 'I can give life but also take life – what a paradox! ... The abortion many years ago has overshadowed our sex life and taken away the right to enjoy it ... I feel hostility towards my husband who pressurised me ... and I have such sad thoughts about it.

(dr)

Time moderates but does not heal all wounds

Some women experience a time of depression when they reach the menopause. It is not unusual for the memory of an abortion that took place 20 or 25 years ago to come to the surface and cause feelings of deep depression and grief.

(dr)

Insight and maturity after pastoral counselling or confession

In a therapy or confessional situation, an individual has the opportunity to speak openly and frankly to a psychiatrist or a Catholic priest about the problems that are troubling them. Women often consult a psychiatrist later in life (perhaps 20 years or more after the abortion), whereas confession to a Catholic priest may take place soon after an abortion.

Confession versus pastoral counselling/therapy

They come to confession in order to have their sins forgiven by God, and they come for pastoral counselling in order to talk to a listening and understanding person – a doctor or a priest.

(cp)

Reconciliation and forgiveness

They accuse themselves of a crime against God and of having betrayed their own values. I have had only a few cases soon after the abortion. Often I have seen women in church who suddenly stop going for Holy Communion. After many, many years they tell the whole story in a confession ... they then feel a sense of reconciliation and are set free!

(cp)

Relief obtained by communication

Through communication they often get a new insight into the problem and the realities of life, and most of them obtain relief from the guilty feelings and gain more strength to continue their lives.

(dr)

Reflection about abortion and the importance of communication

The study involved only a small group of respondents, compared with the large numbers of abortions that are performed (over 30 000 each year in Sweden). The experiences of contact with women after abortion, over a period of 10–40 years, were summarised and described for the researcher not by the women themselves, but by psychiatrists and Catholic priests.

The phenomenological method[9] enables us 'to go back to the things themselves', to discover and analyse the narratives from people's lived experiences. Without compromising professional confidentiality, the psychiatrists and Catholic priests were able to share parts of a summarised rich domain of knowledge from their contacts with women who had had an abortion.

After the interview data had been analysed, the meaning units were grouped according to five themes (*see* Figure 6.1). One of the aims of the study was to find out whether long-term problems may occur after abortion. In most of the interviews it was obvious that the narratives described long-term consequences of abortion for some women and men.

Guilt and shame

In this study many women, and sometimes also their male partners, appeared to experience guilt and shame over a period of years. This might be accounted for by their religious background in some cases, or by depressive tendencies or psychiatric disorder in others. Clearly there are patients at risk, for whom special counselling or therapy is needed, or at least a follow-up to assess their ability to cope with their experience of abortion.

A Canadian study by Ney and Wickett[14] showed that a woman with psychiatric problems related to abortion may not always link her problems to the abortion itself. As one psychiatrist in the study said:

> ... she used different metaphors for her trauma ... but as soon as she mentioned the word 'abortion', it was like peeling an onion, to open up and remove layer after layer of repressed sadness and despair.

This took place 12–15 years after the abortion, and it highlights the special needs of the woman for counselling after the abortion. In accordance with many research studies [2,8,15] most women want to speak about their abortion if they are given the opportunity to do so. It is also emphasised that in the woman's anamneses the abortion must be brought up (or written down), out of consideration for herself.

Effect of family influences

The possibility of an elective abortion being performed because, for example, the fetus is of the 'wrong' gender is one of the negative side-effects of medical and technological progress. Many respondents described how, for religious or cultural reasons, the husband had pressurised his wife to have an abortion if the fetus was female, in the hope that subsequently at least one boy would be born.

Another problem occurs when the male partner ignores or refuses to try to understand the situation. For example, he might say 'Do what you want.' As one Catholic priest commented, *'this in fact amounts to deceit or guile ... the exact opposite of love!'* Trybulski[14] and other researchers show from their studies that many adverse physical as well as psychological effects were experienced by women who felt a lack of support by their partner or other relatives or close friends.

Effect of social influences

The pregnant woman must be given time to reflect on her situation before she decides whether or not to have an abortion. For many women and their partners this is a very difficult and anxious time so long as there are two alternatives. Many studies have described the poor quality of our current information and counselling programmes.[4,14–17] Both the psychiatrists and the Catholic priests in the study described in this chapter discussed the need for an obligatory consultation before the woman decides whether to terminate her pregnancy. One doctor said:

> I felt that those women found it very helpful during quite a difficult and time-consuming decision-making process to be given time to discuss the problem and to reflect on it, and thus in some respects to work through the problem.

Memories and sadness

As mentioned above, many of the summarised experiences of women in the study referred to long-term memories and sadness after abortion:

> One woman said, 12 years after her abortion, 'I have not only damaged and killed a baby, but I have also damaged my own life.'

Ashton[7] reported that 5% of women had long-term severe psychiatric disturbances following abortion, and that individuals especially at risk were those with a previous psychiatric or abnormal obstetric history, or with physical indications for abortion, and those who expressed ambivalence about having an abortion. Other studies involving larger samples of women who had undergone abortion have reported that long-term negative consequences are rare.[6,7,14,15]

Insight and maturity after pastoral counselling or confession

If women are provided with information and counselling at any stage after confirmation of an unwanted pregnancy, they are often able to gain new insights into the problem, their feelings of guilt are lifted, their strength is renewed, and they feel a sense of reconciliation and are set free.

References

1 World Health Organization. *Family Planning Legislation.* Copenhagen: Euro Reports and Studies, 1985.

2 Bengtsson Agostino M, Rum A & Wahlberg V. Women and men in the abortion situation. *Eur J Public Health.* 1993; **3:** 254–8.

3 Holmberg LI & Wahlberg V. The process of decision-making on abortion: a grounded theory study of young men in Sweden. *J Adolesc Health.* 2000; **26:** 230–34.

4 Benson J, Leonard AH, Winkler J, Wolf M & McLaurin KE. *Meeting Women's Needs for Post-Abortion Family Planning: Framing the questions.* Carrboro, NC, Ipas, USA. 1992.

5 SFS. *Abortlagen (the Abortion Act)* (Swedish text). In: The Swedish Statute Book, 1974. SFS, *The Swedish Statute Manual* (Swedish text), Wilow K, Liber AB, Stockholm. 2000: 334.

6 Lapple M. Abortion on demand. Descriptive and quantitative study of psychological and psychosocial aspects. *Contracept Fertil Sex.* 1994; **22:** 117–22.

7 Ashton JR. The psychosocial outcome of induced abortion. *Br J Obstet Gynaecol.* 1980; **87:** 1115–22.

8 Wahlberg V. A phenomenological study of post-abortion syndrome in Sweden. Interviews with psychiatric doctors and Catholic priests. *Int Nurs Perspect.* 2001; **1:** 105–11.

9 Husserl E. *Phenomenology and the Crisis of Philosophy: philosophy as rigorous science, and philosophy and the crisis of European Man* (trans. Q Lauer). New York: Harper & Row, 1965.

10 Beck CT. Phenomenology: its use in nursing research. *Int J Nurs Stud.* 1994; **31:** 499–510.

11 Oiler C. The phenomenological approach in nursing research. *Nurs Res.* 1982; **3:** 178–81.

12 Burns N & Grove S. *The Practice of Nursing Research.* Philadelphia, PA: Saunders Company, 1993.

13 Spiegelberg H. *The Phenomenological Movement. Volume 2.* The Hague: Martinus Nijhoff, 1965.

14 Trybulski, JA. The long-term phenomenon of women's post abortion experiences. *Western J Nurs Res.* 2005; **27:** 559–76.

15 Goebel, P. A comparison of the psychosocial status of 125 abortion patients before and after the termination of pregnancy. *Z Psychosom Med Psychoanal.* 1984; **30:** 270–81.

16 Bengtsson Agostino M. Information needs among Italian abortion patients. *Gynecol Obstet Invest.* 1997; **43:** 84–8.

17 Holmberg LI & Wahlberg V. The staff's views regarding young men involved in decisions on abortion: preliminary information from a study of Outpatient Clinics for Adolescents in Sweden. *Gynecol Obstet Invest.* 1999; **47:** 177–81.

Chapter 7

Different conditions of life

Vivian Wahlberg

Introduction

In order to convey some idea of how much life in Sweden has changed and certainly also improved in many respects during the last 100 years, this chapter will start with an overview of relevant legislation that has come into force since the beginning of the twentieth century. These are very important milestones that are of particular significance for the family and the young generation. Modern lifestyles and their problems and potential are also discussed, and the chapter ends with some reflections on young people's longing to feel needed and loved.

Looking back

Then and now: some milestones in Sweden in the twentieth century

At a public health conference in 1985, a professor of sociology presented the results of a study of different trends in society and the public health sector in Sweden. This lecture gave me many fresh perspectives and a new understanding of the life that we create for ourselves. Over 20 years have passed since then, but I still have the conference folder on my bookshelf and often look back on the following notes.

- Between 1918 and 1921 the democratisation process started in Sweden.
- In 1921 Swedish women gained the right to vote.
- In 1935, maternity welfare and antenatal care were introduced.
- In 1938, the special law relating to contraceptives (which had made it punishable to demonstrate and give public information about contraceptives and advice about their use) was abrogated.
- In 1938, the first Abortion Act came into force, permitting termination of pregnancy on three different grounds – medico-social, humanitarian and eugenic.
- The 1940s generation began to break with old traditions, and there were changes in disciplinary issues, especially for children and young people.
- In 1946, a socio-medical change was made to the Abortion Act, namely that a woman no longer needed to show signs of illness or weakness in order to have an abortion granted.

- In 1948, the law was changed so that it was no longer possible to dismiss a woman from her employment because she was pregnant.
- In 1948, the national child benefit was introduced.
- In the 1950s the first real consumer society began to emerge, the first teenage consumers came on the scene, and there was a new breakthrough in the mass media (television, electronics, etc.).
- In the 1960s, student movements were formed and some mass rebellions took place. A debate about gender roles began, and the role of women and their liberation, independence and equality with men were asserted.
- In 1960, 40% of women were in employment. A report about national day nurseries was presented, and day care under community management began to take form.
- In 1962, the oral contraceptive pill was introduced and the use of contraception in general by society increased.
- In 1963, the thalidomide disaster led to another new indication for termination of pregnancy.
- In 1964, the intrauterine device (IUD) was introduced. Sexual activity in young people was increasingly accepted, and the Abortion Act became more liberal.
- From 1965, a person could be found guilty of rape even if it occurred within marriage.
- From 1965, the frequency of marriage began to decline, and the concept of unmarried couples living together began to be accepted.
- In 1970, around 90% of married couples had lived together before their marriage.
- In 1971, separate taxation of husbands and wives was initiated.
- In 1973, a marriage law came into force that made it easier to obtain a divorce.
- In 1974, a regulation concerning parental leave was introduced, which gave parents the right to take time off work after the birth of a child. At the same time parental education was initiated.
- In 1974 a new Abortion Act was introduced, which came into force in January 1975.
- In the 1980s, norms and traditional values started to disintegrate. There were debates about young people, particularly about their anxiety and their feelings of having lost their way in life.

The above list could be much longer. Since the early 1990s, questions of equal opportunity for both sexes and the other issue of gender perspectives/gender gap have been frequently debated, and the position of women has been further strengthened. At the same time, however, a number of setbacks have been noted. For example, in many countries prostitution has been legalised, which raises the question of whether, in a democracy, it should be possible to 'buy' women and children like any other commodity.[1]

The so-called *sex purchase law* (which is so far unique to Sweden) was introduced in 1999. It has been defined as follows:

To buy, or try to buy, sexual services is from 1 January 1999 a criminal offence that is punishable with a fine or up to six months in prison.[1]

This is an important stand against countries that are considering or have already introduced legalisation of prostitution, and highlights the fact that Sweden regards this practice as a serious form of oppression of women.[1]

Discussion of legislation against the physical and/or sexual abuse of women dates back to the thirteenth century, but women still suffer in this respect. Through the 1999 legislation relating to abuse of women, the Swedish Parliament has tried to stop repeated physical and/or sexual abuse by a close or previously close family member or a partner by making this punishable with imprisonment for a minimum of six months and a maximum of six years.[2]

The number of reports of rape and attempted rape has doubled in the last few years. We have read of numerous tragic assaults and rapes in which both the perpetrator and the victim were very young. Everyone has the right to express their own sexuality, but no one has the right to injure or abuse another person.

Sex trafficking (the movement of human beings across geographical borders for sexual purposes) has been prohibited by Swedish law since 1 July 2002. Most commonly it is young girls from Eastern Europe who are brought into Sweden to become prostitutes. However, lack of evidence often makes it difficult to bring to justice 'pimps' and others who sexually abuse these girls. We live in a fairly brutal 'culture of happiness', and the price for this is high. Again I want to refer to the lecture mentioned above, especially with regard to the question of young people's anxiety and their feelings of having lost their way in life.

In summary, it may be said that the Swedish legislation mentioned above has had many positive consequences in terms of establishing social justice at different levels in society. Among other things it has allowed greater emancipation of women, and has considerably improved their general status in Sweden.

The start of different preventive projects

At the end of the twentieth century, society began to contribute more than previously to different forms of collaboration between, for example, the municipality, primary healthcare, schools, social services, club activities and committees for recreational activities. One of the many aims was to prevent the establishment of criminal gangs and to influence young people's early relationships and sexual habits.

More than 30 years ago an intervention project consisting of a 4-year trial was initiated in Gotland, the largest island in Sweden, with a focus on personal relationships among young people and measures to prevent abortion. After the trial had been running for only two years the results showed a 30% reduction in teenage abortions. At the same time there was a tendency for both teenage pregnancies and teenage abortions to occur at older ages, as well as a decrease in the total number of teenage pregnancies.

Another example is the project known as SamS, concerning personal relationships, which was introduced in the late 1980s in a county on the west coast of Sweden (Landstinget i Älvsborg – county council of Älvsborg).[3] The basic aim of the project was to support the role of adults in their contact with young people so as to improve their ability to understand the needs of adolescents and thereby increase the self-esteem of the latter. Adults who work with young people often also need further education about sexuality and relationships, as well as training to improve their ability to meet the needs of adolescents in an effective way. An important additional goal of this project was to reduce the number of teenage abortions.

Several different projects are being conducted in different parts of Sweden with the aim of promoting positive views on sex and relationships and preventing pregnancy and sexually transmitted diseases (especially HIV/AIDS) among young people. The results of these projects indicate the importance of involvement of people from different sectors of society, and of the growth and development of supportive networks. It is also important to set aside days or weeks that are devoted to this particular theme of prevention and support (e.g. with the use of drama on the topic, and parents' meetings).

Evaluation of the above-mentioned project showed that personal relationship issues and sex-related questions dominated different discussions and activities targeted at young people. An awareness of the importance of and need for meaningful meetings for both adolescents and adults was also evident. This is illustrated by the following extract from one interview:[3]

> During a true encounter you make contact with another person and you understand something about that person's thoughts and values. You learn something about yourself and you gain a greater insight into the thoughts and needs of others.

In today's pressurised society, there is seldom enough time or opportunity for real communication between people. However, it is the dialogue close to everyday life that makes it possible to have the deep and meaningful exchange of thoughts which is so important, especially between children and their parents. We therefore need to consider whether our lack of time is due to our self-absorption or whether it is a consequence of the structure and organisation of society and/or the ethos of the time.

There seem to be far too many young people today who have no real contact in their lives, and who therefore experience a great sense of loneliness. They find it difficult to see any meaning in life, and there is a risk that they will try to produce their own meaning through dubious contacts, and behaviours involving sexual risk, drug abuse or even criminality.

Where does the modern individual stand today?

Sexuality, which is a powerful instinct, permeates the lives of most people, and when handled in the right way it is a tremendous resource, providing excitement, pleasure and relaxation, and reducing stress. However, if used in the wrong way it can cause deep emotional wounds and frustration that can lead to verbal aggression and even physical violence against oneself or others. To prevent this, young people need in-depth education about the many dimensions of sexuality as well as the dangers that may result from its mishandling.

Inexplicable tendencies and pain that is difficult to master

Compulsive eating or bulimia

We often read today about teenage girls who have eating disorders and starve themselves or suffer from bulimia, or who cut themselves or cause self-harm in various other ways. For example, in one interview a young girl said *'When I saw the blood oozing out, the anxiety disappeared.'* The important question that must be asked is how and why this situation has arisen. How many unfulfilled expectations and how much mortification and grief lie behind such actions? How often are they a result of relationship difficulties?

Vulvar vestibulitis

In the last few years it has become increasingly common for young women to experience pain in the genitals and vagina that is difficult to treat, with dry and irritated mucous membranes, spontaneous chapping of the mucosa, and inexplicable pain during sexual intercourse.[4] This might be due to lack of foreplay prior to sexual intercourse. This initial phase normally stimulates lubrication, but young people seldom have time for it today. As many girls stated, *'There is no time for foreplay – it all has to happen so quickly!'*

It is calculated that up to 5% of women aged between 20 and 30 years suffer from repeated fungal infections or vulvar pain, so-called *vulvar vestibulitis,* a condition that causes redness and pain of the vestibule of the vagina. Vestibulitis often affects the whole area around the opening of the vagina, but is most commonly seen in the lower region. Many women with this problem suffer physically and emotionally for months or even years with severe pain on pressure (e.g. when riding a bicycle, when horse-riding, when wearing tight-fitting clothes, etc.). Tampon use or sexual intercourse can cause a burning, stinging, irritating or raw sensation in the vestibular area. Many women have seen a number of gynaecologists and have tried several unsuccessful treatments in their search for relief of their symptoms. The exact cause of the condition is unknown, but many studies are currently in progress to attempt to elucidate the underlying cause. Factors such as *'different degrees of stress, sexual dysfunction and/or nervous tension or mental problems, giving rise to symptoms in the vulva'*[5] have been associated with vulvar vestibulitis.

Sexual assault and violence against women

Recently a Nordic investigation involving a total of 3641 women, which was published in the *Lancet* and subsequently in many newspapers, showed that sexual assault and violence against women are considerably more prevalent than had previously been thought to be the case. Furthermore, the study showed that one in six gynaecology patients had experienced sexual assault at some time earlier in their life, and one in ten had been forced to have sex.[6]

Health habits and risk-taking behaviours

A self-administered questionnaire

A relevant factor in this context is the lifestyle of young people today compared with that observed previously. This includes their health habits, their sense of well-being and the different forms of risk-taking behaviour in which they engage. To investigate this, a study was conducted in 1995 on 18-year-old boys in a Swedish upper secondary school in a medium-sized Swedish city.

A self-administered questionnaire was used that included questions on health, health habits and risk-taking behaviour, in order to compare the lifestyles of young men.[7,8] The questionnaire covered domains such as family background, puberty, health, illnesses, academic performance, peer relationships, quality of life, and various forms of behaviour (eating, driving, exercise, sexuality, and use of tobacco, alcohol and illicit drugs).

The questionnaires were completed anonymously by a total of 1175 male respondents, and were then analysed. The respondents were divided into three groups:

1   those who had never had sexual intercourse
2   those who were sexually active but had not been involved in a pregnancy
3   those who had been involved in a pregnancy.

Some selected results from the study

More than 50% of the respondents had had sexual intercourse, and around 5% had also been involved in a pregnancy. As the study was only conducted in one municipality, the results need to be interpreted with some caution.

The boys who had had sexual intercourse tended to be more likely to have come from broken homes compared with the other boys, particularly if they had also been involved in a pregnancy. Furthermore, a higher proportion of the boys from group 3, who had caused a pregnancy, had experienced early puberty and believed that they were regarded as older than their biological age.

In addition, the results showed that the boys in group 1, who had not had sexual intercourse, were more successful at school and were less likely to play truant than those who had experience of intercourse. Furthermore, the boys in group 1 had been injured less often than those in groups 2 and 3, and had less often been hospitalised as a result of accidents.

Some other tendencies were also evident. For example, the boys in group 3, who had been involved in a pregnancy, were much more likely to have considered suicide than those in the other two groups. The boys in group 3 also used seat belts in cars less often than the other boys, and they had more erratic eating habits (e.g. they seldom had breakfast) and were more likely to use alcohol and illicit drugs. With regard to risk-taking behaviour, the boys in group 3 more often got into fights, smoked and used anabolic steroids (which are known to cause physical and mental harm).

As expected, the respondents in group 3 who had been involved in a pregnancy used contraceptives less often. These boys were also more likely to have had sexually transmitted diseases than the boys in group 1. The boys in group 3 had had several more sexual partners than those in groups 1 and 2. Furthermore, the respondents in group 3 were more likely to have been sexually abused by adults than the boys in the other two groups.

New life patterns

We are living in a time when one new development follows closely on another. For example, by hormone treatment and/or surgery even the laws of nature can be challenged, from age limits for parenthood to attempts to make our bodies look more beautiful by plastic surgery. Most of this seems to be related to our sexual and reproductive needs and ability. For instance, attempts to increase the power of attraction through enlargement of the breasts or penis, face-lifts, operations on the eyelids, lip surgery, and so on, are fairly recent phenomena in human history. Among young people it is also increasingly common to be tattooed or to have one's ears, nose, lips or other body parts pierced. This preoccupation with an attractive appearance is in sharp contrast to the peasant society of old (not a time to which we would want to return!).

The view of parenthood is changing

As a result of research and technological advances, there is now a much greater likelihood that couples will be able to have children (e.g. by egg and sperm donation, embryo transfer, *in-vitro* fertilisation (IVF), and so on). The approximately half a million Swedish people who are suffering from infertility have three main alternatives:

1   to seek medical assistance and treatment for the problem
2   to apply for adoption
3   to accept a life without children.[9]

In many parts of the world there are ongoing major developments in the context and timing of childbirth. It was recently reported that as a result of treatment by a physician in Italy, a 58-year-old woman had successfully become pregnant, and that after receiving hormone treatment throughout the pregnancy she gave birth to a child despite her relatively advanced age. Newspaper reports bore headlines such as '*Shall grandma be mother again?*'

In many states in the USA it has for many years been possible to pay a surrogate mother to produce a child. Another report, from England, stated that '*One twin was aborted during early pregnancy.*' This was because the parents considered that it would be too demanding to take care of two children at the same time.

The Internet, television and the media: problems and potential

In recent years the Internet, email and computer games have become commonplace in our homes and in society in general. Young people now have almost limitless access not only to a vast wealth of information and knowledge, but also to numerous dubious opportunities through the circle of contacts that can be made around the world in almost any sphere of interest. Many parents do not appear to have adequate control over their children's access to and surfing on the Internet.

In Sweden, the Knowledge Foundation has a website devoted to information and communication technology (ICT) in education. The purpose of this site is to promote the use of ICT as a tool in the education of young people. Over the years it has become a lively and extremely active site visited by thousands of individuals across Sweden, who can share their knowledge and experience, discuss problems, and so on.

In 2003, the results of a research study conducted by the Knowledge Foundation were published in a Swedish newspaper.[10] The study included 4700 children
aged between 9 and 16 years from Denmark, Ireland, Iceland, Norway and
Sweden. The results showed that children and adolescents visited websites that
were quite different from those that their parents believed they were using.
Furthermore, the accounts given by adults were not consistent with the children's
answers. For example, 80% of the parents stated that they usually sat with their
child at the computer, whereas 70% of the children said that their mother or
father never sat with them at the computer. In addition, the study showed that
nine out of ten teenagers used chat-rooms on the Internet, and that a third of
these young people had sometimes been threatened, frightened or humiliated
during their Internet contacts. There can obviously be serious risks involved in
children's arrangements to meet people with whom they have made contact via
the Internet.

Many newspapers have recently highlighted the issue of children aged 11–12
years who, according to investigations in southern Europe, watch pornographic
films on the Internet on a daily basis. Perhaps pornography should not be rejected
completely, but among children of this age it is highly inappropriate to arouse
incipient lust and curiosity in this way. Moreover, some 'hard' pornography is so
coarse and brutal that it can completely distort and impair the normal development of a young person's sexual identity.

As was discussed earlier in this book (*see* Chapter 3), many adolescents have
described their disillusionment when they imitated what they had heard and
seen on television, in films and in the media, or what they had heard through
friends, and how they betrayed their own ideals by engaging in casual relationships that had no lasting value and gave rise to feelings of degradation and
self-disgust.

However, the Internet also has many positive aspects. It can supply news and
information, convey messages, provide valuable knowledge and give global perspectives to which we have never previously had access. Children and adolescents
in need of adult support can also obtain help and advice via the Internet.

In Sweden there is a Children's Ombudsman. The head of the Office of
the Children's Ombudsman[11] has described in a press release a new site on the
Internet, named *Hello!*, which can be reached via its website.[12] It offers useful tips
on what to do if, for example, a young person is unhappily in love, is being
victimised, or is worried about their parents' quarrelling. It also provides information on children's rights.[12] In Sweden there are several other websites and
telephone numbers for young people who need someone to talk to because they
are in a difficult or critical situation.

Earlier in this chapter I referred to milestones during the twentieth century and
the debates that took place, particularly about young people, their anxiety and
their sense of having lost their way in life. Everything today seems to be moving
at a tremendous speed. There is a vast flow of information, and rapid changes are
taking place both in the local environment and internationally. In view of this, it
is not surprising that many young people lose their footing and question their
own direction in life.

In a Stockholm evening newspaper, a chief editor reflected on the future
that we are creating, and stated '*It is easy to make someone pregnant, but not so easy to
be a parent.*' Referring to the many cases of personal injury and murder during

the previous summer, he continued his reflection about the background of a young man being held in custody:[13]

> Did he ever, as a child, have a book in his hand?
> Did he at any time go fishing with his father?
> Did anybody at any time make eye contact with him or listen to him?
> Did he ever have a teddy bear? Was he ever cuddled?
> Did he feel a sense of security, knowing that he was loved?

And the strong society of which we are so proud and that we still believe to be world class – was it willing to help for long enough, while there was still time and hope?

- What did the school do?
- What did the healthcare system do?
- Did anyone sound the alarm?

Politicians and representatives of schools, churches, social services and others all highlight the need for a stable social network, safe and secure adult contacts, and the ability of young people who are in a relationship to share questions of vital importance with their partner. How in today's stressful society will we find the time to address the questions and the longing of children and young people to feel needed and loved?

References

1 Häggström-Nordin E. The effects of legalization of prostitution (Swedish text). *Jordemodern.*, January/February 2003.

2 The Swedish criminal (penal) code against violation of a woman's integrity, Chapter 4 (Swedish text). The Swedish Parliament, Stockholm, (Law 1999:845).

3 Halldén B-M & Edgren L. The project on sexuality and relationship (SamS): evaluation of a Swedish municipality district project (Swedish text). *Socialvetenskaplig tidskrift.* 2000; **4**: 346–60.

4 Gustavsson L. *Inexplicable Pain During Coitus. An interview study about connection style and affect, shame and sexuality among young women with inexplicable pain during coitus* (Swedish text). Stockholm: Swedish Institute of Cognitive Psychotherapy, 2002.

5 Rylander E. *Leading researchers in Norden on vulva illnesses* (Swedish text). Advertisement from Mediaplanet, Stockholm, 2003.

6 Holender R. Sexual assault experienced by one in six gynaecology patients. Earlier abuses are documented in a new report (Swedish text). *Svenska Dagbladet*, 4 July 2003.

7 Berg-Kelly K. Normative developmental behaviour with implications for health and health promotion among adolescents: a Swedish cross-sectional survey. *Acta Paediatr.* 1995; **84**: 278–88.

8 Holmberg L & Berg-Kelly K. Health, health-compromising behaviour, sexuality and involvement in pregnancy among 18-year-old Swedish males: a cross-sectional survey. *Acta Paediatr.* 2002; **91**: 838–43.

9 Arfs M. All alternatives ought to be inspected (Swedish text). *Jordemodern, The Swedish Midwife Journal*, April 2003.

10 Agebäck AK. Children live their own life on the Net (summary of a study from the Swedish Knowledge Foundation, formerly the Våldskildringsrådet) (Swedish text). *Svenska Dagbladet*, 23 May 2003.

11 Nyman L. Press release from the Barnombudsman (Swedish text). *Svenska Dagbladet*, 3 July 2003.

12 Hello! (website for children and young people in Sweden); www.bo.se.

13 Ekman P. *We Get the World We Create Together* (Swedish text). Stockholm: CITY. 29 September 2003.

Chapter 8

Epilogue: a final reflection from an ethical perspective

António Barbosa da Silva

Introduction

The previous chapters of this book were mainly descriptive. In contrast, this chapter is written from an ethically normative perspective that can be explained as follows. It includes an analysis of some relevant moral problems that are raised by the rest of the book. The main purpose of the analysis is to highlight the moral responsibility shared by all of those individuals, groups and organisations that are involved in an induced abortion. The most important of these are the pregnant woman who chooses abortion (the *aborting woman*), her partner, her parents or significant others, the healthcare professionals who perform the abortion (the *abortionists*), the society in which the woman lives, and the state (represented by the Swedish National Board of Health and Welfare).

Throughout the analysis the underlying notion is that the aborting woman may be harmed in two different ways with regard to abortion ethics, which must be considered as ethically unjust when her responsibility for choosing abortion is compared to that of the other above-mentioned individuals, groups and organisations. Thus she can feel remorse, guilt, shame and angst* partly because she has chosen abortion, and partly as a result of the actions of the abortionists in inducing the abortion.

This brief ethical reflection was inspired and motivated by the new knowledge and insight gained from the results of the investigations described in the previous chapters. The material for analysis mainly concerns some relevant aspects of abortion and its various causes which were not addressed in depth in the previous chapters, and which therefore require further ethical reflection. Against this background, this chapter is not only an epilogue, as its title indicates, but also a relevant although brief ethical consideration of the intricate moral issues raised by the book as a whole.

Fundamental ethical themes that are to be highlighted here include ethical norms and values, and the concepts of freedom, responsibility and human dignity, and worth, guilt and shame. We hope as more aspects of the complex phenomenon of abortion are clarified, and as more people (especially pregnant women) become aware of this clarification, that the women who must make a decision about abortion will be better equipped to do so.

---

*In this context the word 'angst' is philosophically more appropriate than the word 'anxiety.'

The themes that are discussed here and in the other chapters indicate that abortion is a complex phenomenon that requires a thorough assessment, if an ethical evaluation of all the different aspects of the performance or inducement of an abortion is to be made.[1]

The precondition for an ethical assessment of abortion: a holistic approach

This book offers two types of knowledge and insight. The first type is about how the pregnant woman who opts for abortion and her partner experience the negative consequences of the abortion. The other type of knowledge that the book indirectly addresses concerns the lack of a comprehensive analysis and ethical assessment of the complex phenomenon of abortion. This lack of knowledge is identified in discussions of abortion and its causes, as our investigations have shown, and it is also confirmed by international studies on abortion.[2]

With regard to the first type of knowledge and insight (about the experiences of aborting women), we shall briefly analyse the different factors involved, an understanding of which may shed considerable light on the actual or assumed moral responsibility of each of the above-mentioned agents, who are involved either in the aborting woman's decision making about abortion, or in inducing the abortion.

From this perspective we shall analyse abortion as a complex phenomenon that requires a holistic ethical approach to the decision to have an abortion as well as to the inducement of the procedure. We believe that such an approach has relevant consequences for the attribution of moral responsibility to the agents implicated in the decision to have an abortion, as well as in the inducement of the abortion.

To illustrate another aspect of abortion, we shall present an ethical appraisal of the fate of the aborted fetus with regard to its moral consequences. Some ways of handling the aborted fetus tend to cause or incite guilt in the aborting woman and others. We shall therefore ethically evaluate some of the ways of handling the aborted fetus that tend to cause feelings of guilt in the above-mentioned agents, especially the aborting woman.

In addition, we shall discuss the complexity of the abortion phenomenon that actualises a holistic approach to abortion, with the latter seen as a moral action. This approach has relevance for the attribution of moral responsibility to the various moral agents who are voluntarily involved in the action. We shall start by clarifying the concept of moral responsibility.

Moral responsibility and its necessary conditions

Our enquiry indicates that sometimes too much responsibility is attributed to the aborting woman with regard to her choice of abortion. She is without doubt the most prominent agent implicated in an induced abortion, as it is she who carries the fetus and it is to her alone that the law of free abortion gives the right to either terminate or continue her pregnancy. However, these facts by themselves cannot constitute a cogent argument for attributing all of the responsibility related to abortion to her, solely because she chooses abortion. The various motives and reasons for her choice, as well as the various agents implicated in such a choice, should be considered in close relation to her presumed responsibility.[3]

Therefore her partner may have some responsibility, or as much as she does, depending on whether and how he influences her decision making. Also the society in which the woman lives, which consists of various agents who in different ways and for various reasons may be involved in an abortion case, may have some responsibility (e.g. for the fate of the fetus, and for the life and health of the aborting woman and her partner after the abortion). We also maintain that abortion should not be the only means of resolving the conflict of interests, values or moral dilemmas that may be experienced by a pregnant woman.[4]

However, before we discuss the distribution of accountability, it is relevant to analyse some of the criteria that are necessary for a person to fulfil if he or she is to be morally responsible for what he or she does.

Free will, deliberation and choice, and freedom of action

The concept of moral or ethical responsibility is closely related to the concept of freedom or autonomy, which implies that without autonomy there can be no moral responsibility. However, some controversial issues arise in this context, which have been discussed for over 2000 years, throughout the history of ethics. For example:

1 What is meant by autonomy (free will, free choice and free decision or action)?*
2 Under what circumstances is human action free? In other words, is human action ultimately free or is it determined by the laws of nature in the same way that natural events are determined by the laws of nature?[5]

As an illustration of these issues, we can say that when someone throws a stone up into the air (a human action), after some time it will turn downwards (a natural event) because of the law of gravitation, a law of nature that is an integral part of natural order. Thus human action presupposes human free will as its cause, whereas a natural event presupposes a natural law as its cause.

The fact that human beings are free means that they have *free will* (i.e. the capacity to think or discern the existence or possibility of different courses of action). Freedom of will is the basis of *deliberation* and *freedom of choice*, which is the capacity to choose one particular action from a range of possible actions. In order for people to be morally responsible or blamed for what they do, they must be free in these two different but closely related senses. They must also be free in a third sense, namely to decide and act without coercion, which means to have a real option of performing the chosen action. Harald Ofstad has defined the freedom of decision or action as 'the power to act otherwise.'[6] Freedom in this threefold sense is a necessary condition if people are to be morally responsible for their actions and for their experience of guilt or remorse, and for their wrongdoings to be judged as genuine.

---

*Kant identifies free will or autonomy with 'practical reason.' (cf. Heubel F & Biller-Andorno N. The contribution of Kantian moral theory to contemporary medical ethics: a critical analysis. *Med Healthcare Philos*. 2005; **7**: 5–18.)

Although our investigation does not primarily address the aborting woman's freedom, according to the threefold sense described above, perhaps the pro-abortion choice of those women who experience feelings of guilt and angst after abortion can be explained by the fact that they did not have 'the power to act otherwise' when they opted for abortion as the best thing to do in their situation. In other words, they did not have freedom of decision. They might have had freedom to discern various alternative courses of action, but it was not possible for them to decide and act otherwise. One of the reasons for this might be that their knowledge of different aspects of abortion was deficient. Perhaps their parents, teachers and 'significant others' who had been responsible for their education taught them nothing or very little about the psychological, existential, moral and religious aspects of induced abortion. Perhaps they did not receive any teaching about sexual ethics, family ethics and their basic human, social and economic rights. Perhaps if during their deliberations for or against abortion they had thought that their psychological and existential suffering after abortion might be greater than their happiness and economic welfare, they might have acted otherwise. Furthermore, perhaps if they had read, for example, some of the writings of Dostoyevsky, Tolstoy, Kierkegaard or Frankl about the meaning of life and suffering, moral responsibility, guilt, angst, remorse and despair, they would have acquired the knowledge necessary to enable them to act differently (i.e. to decide against abortion). In addition, in many cases of induced abortion, the pregnant woman has no choice. As one woman declared, *'If just one of my friends had said ''I'll be there for you,'' I could have made it.'*[7] That is, she could have had her baby.*

Freedom of action as the power to act otherwise

Given that freedom of decision or action means 'to have it in one's power to act otherwise',[†] the lack of power to act otherwise that may sometimes be experienced should humble people and make them willing to share the collective responsibility that society has for each case of induced abortion. If we are aware that other people may not always have freedom of action, then we should refrain from 'casting the first stone'[8] – that is, we should not judge others. If they did not have the power to act otherwise, then they were not free in the threefold sense defined above. Therefore they cannot be morally responsible for their actions.

Furthermore, it should be emphasised that the fact that the aborting woman sometimes experiences feelings of guilt does not necessarily mean that she is actually guilty and morally responsible implying that she acted immorally by having an abortion. Her feeling of guilt may be a false one. Rollo May[9] distinguishes between false guilt and a genuine existential or ontological experience of guilt. The latter, but not the former, is an integral part of the nature of man, and is essential for a normal healthy life. Rollo May characterises existential or ontological guilt as follows:

---

* For an account of the physiological problems caused by induced abortion, see Moreau C, Kaminski M, Ancel PY *et al*. Previous induced abortions and the risk of very preterm delivery: results of the EPIPAGE study. *Int J Obstet Gynecol*. 2005; **112**: 430–37.

† Cf. with Ofstad H. *Responsibility and Action. Introduction to moral philosophical problems* (Swedish text). Stockholm: Prisma, 1982: 203.

... ontological guilt has, among others, these characteristics. First, everyone participates in it. No one of us fails to some extent to distort the reality of his fellow men, and no one completely fulfils his own potential ... Second, ontological guilt does not come from cultural prohibitions, ... it is rooted in the fact of self-awareness. Ontological guilt does not consist of I am guilty because I violate potential prohibitions, but arises from the fact that I can see myself as the one who can choose or fail to choose ... Third, ontological guilt is not to be confused with morbid or neurotic guilt. ... Fourth, ontological guilt does not lead to symptom formation, but has constructive effect in the personality ...[9]

According to May, choice is intrinsically related to the experience of existential or ontological guilt, which is a fundamental human characteristic. Therefore it should be clearly distinguished from both the pathological feeling of guilt and the authentic moral guilt that only results from a voluntarily performed action which is morally wrong. In other words, moral guilt is closely linked to moral responsibility. One can also experience a feeling of *false* guilt – 'morbid or neurotic guilt',* as May explains it.[9] A woman who has undergone an induced abortion can experience all three kinds of guilt. She therefore needs help to discern which of them is genuine – that is, which is caused by her moral responsibility, which is existential, and which is false guilt. To handle each one of these kinds of guilt appropriately, one needs different kinds of help.

The basis for judging what is morally right or wrong

To illustrate how a normative ethical theory functions as an ethical basis or criterion for judging the rightness or wrongness of an action, let us start with a concrete example. There are at least four ways of answering the question '*Is an induced abortion a right or wrong action?*'

1 An induced abortion is a type of action that is always morally wrong.[10]
2 To induce abortion is morally right if, and only if, its consequences are beneficial to the happiness and/or welfare of as many people as possible, including the aborting woman.
3 To induce abortion is morally right if, and only if, its consequences are beneficial for the aborting woman alone.
4 Abortion is a morally right action if one chooses or induces it on the basis of a good motive or a good moral character.

These four different ways of assessing the moral rightness or wrongness of an action – in this case abortion – illustrate the application of four different normative ethical theories to four different answers to the same question. We shall now consider the ethical theories underlying the four answers given above, which can also be viewed as four ethical assessments of abortion.

---

* May further maintains that '*neurotic guilt is the end product of enforced normal ontological anxiety.*'[9] One can experience remorse if one does not fulfil one's moral obligation or duty. Cf. Hare RM. *Moral Thinking*. Oxford: Oxford University Press, 1981: 29.

Moral assessment of abortion based on four ethical theories

Answer 1 in the above list is made according to the normative ethical theory known as *deontology* (or more precisely, *rule deontology*). The person who argues according to answer 2 is using the normative theory known as *utilitarianism,* which is one form of consequence ethics, whereas answer 3 results from the application of another form of consequence ethics known as *ethical egoism*. This theory states that an action is right if, and only if, its consequences are beneficial for the welfare of the person who performs it. The fundamental principle of utilitarianism is utility, according to which an action is right if, and only if, it maximises human welfare. Answer 4 results from the application of the ethical theory known as the ethics of *virtue* or *character and ideals*.

All normative ethical theories have some drawbacks. One of the weaknesses of rule deontology, which follows strict rules, is that two or more rules can conflict with each other and thus give rise to an ethical dilemma. The latter is a conflict of moral obligations such that whatever choice is made from among the possible or available courses of action, it will lead to a wrong action. For example, rule (i), '*always* tell the truth', can conflict with rule (ii), '*never* harm or kill a human being.' This can occur when telling the truth will have as its consequence the harming or killing of someone. Another example of a dilemma may arise, for example, when a medical doctor is using rule (ii) in a situation in which he has to perform a Caesarean section with the intention of saving the lives of both the mother and the child. He or she will face a moral dilemma if the operation necessarily leads to the death of at least one of them. To choose not to operate will be worse, because both lives may be lost. To avoid or solve this type of dilemma – created by rule deontology – the moral agents should *not* rigidly follow ethical rules and always apply them according to rule deontology. They must also use consequence ethics, virtue ethics or ideals, or intuition to prioritise the rule that they should obey in the situation, in order to solve the dilemma. Consequence ethics, but not rule deontology, allows the moral agent to choose the least harmful action of two or more harmful actions. He may solve the first dilemma described above, for example, by lying in order to save life, whereas to solve the second dilemma he may choose to operate with the hope of saving one life, presumably that of the mother. Consequence ethics can help to solve a dilemma because it allows the consequences of two or more actions to be compared with one another. This is not the case with rule deontology, which applies each rule absolutely and without exception. However, a fundamental drawback of consequence ethics is that no action can be right in itself. Whether an action is right or wrong always depends on its beneficial or harmful consequences. These are not given but subjectively calculated by the person who performs the action.

The distinctive feature of consequence ethics is the overarching principle that the end justifies the means. Ethical egoism, as a form of consequence ethics, cannot constitute the foundation of social ethics because if all people adhered to it, there would be a war of 'everyone against everyone.'[11]

The weakness of the ethics of virtue or character and ideals is that the good intention and motive of the agent is not always sufficient to determine the rightness of his or her action. In addition, given the fact that intention and motive vary from one person to another, there is no independent and reliable inter-subjective criterion for distinguishing good intentions and motives from bad ones.

In order to avoid the weaknesses or limitations of each of the four ethical theories, it is possible and indeed advisable, in certain situations, to combine the advantages of each of them so that they can supplement one another. For example, in some situations it is logically possible to combine aspects of deontology with aspects of consequence ethics and aspects of the ethics of character or virtue and ideals. One would perform an action according to deontology because it is right in itself and it is one's moral obligation do so, according to consequence ethics because it leads to beneficial consequences for as many people as possible (with regard to their welfare or happiness), and according to the ethics of character or virtue and ideals because one has a good motive and intends to do what is good (cf. the virtue of benevolence). Thus one would do what is right for the sake of its rightness, at the same time one would consider the welfare of as many people as possible, and finally one would also use virtue and ideals to promote the common welfare.[12] Actions that in certain circumstances may allow for such a combination of ethical theories include, for example, those that fall under the following obligations:

- 'One ought to tell the truth'
- 'One should not kill an innocent person'
- 'One ought to help people in need.'

By combining some aspects of two or more of the four ethical theories, one embraces 'methodological and theoretical pluralism.'

Those who are against abortion (pro-life supporters) generally argue against it using rule deontology after the manner of Kant.[13] In contrast, those who defend free abortion, according to law, argue from the point of view of consequence ethics (utilitarianism or ethical egoism).[14] The difference between the two standpoints can be explained in the light of what follows.

Morality and ethics, one's view of life and one's view of human beings and their interrelationships

If one intends to argue that certain normative ethics are better than others, one must refer to a given view or concept of the human race, which must be justified or defended in terms of a given view of life (implicit in one's philosophy of life, religion, ideology or culture). In any view of life, there is always an explicitly or implicitly stated view of reality, and given moral or ethical values.[15] The relationship between the concept of life (philosophy of life), the concept of the human race and the concept of morality and ethics can be illustrated as shown in Figure 8.1.

What is morality and what is ethics?

Morality and ethics deal with *norms* (right and wrong) and *values* (good and bad). The term *morality* usually refers to how people take into consideration norms and values in their attitudes and behaviours in real life. The term *ethics* is more commonly used to refer to a philosophical reflection about the moral life.[16] There is no doubt that in real life people in fact continually evaluate their own lives, behaviour and attitudes in terms of right and wrong, and good and bad.

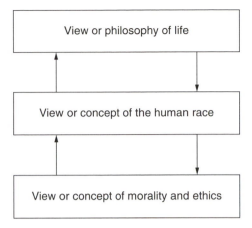

Figure 8.1 The relationship between the concept or view of life (philosophy of life), the concept of the human race, and the concept of morality and ethics. The upward-pointing arrows denote 'is the grounds of' and the downward-pointing arrows denote 'is deducible from'.

An ethical reflection on how people live a moral life aims to answer the following question: 'What is the best way of conducting and evaluating our lives, attitudes and behaviours in terms of right and wrong, and good and bad?' Ethics also deals with definitions of *right, good, moral obligation or duty, responsibility, shame*, etc., as well as the relationship between morality and other domains of human experience, such as religion, aesthetics, metaphysics, etc. It is beyond the scope of this book to discuss all of these issues here, and for a more detailed account of the differences between morality and ethics we refer the reader to the relevant literature.[17]

The relationship between ethical norms and values can be illustrated by the following example. The rule that 'One ought to tell the truth' is a norm expressed by the sentence as a whole. However, this norm contains an ethical value, namely 'truth'. Moreover, the norm 'One ought to respect other people's autonomy, dignity and worth' contains the ethical values 'autonomy', 'dignity' and 'worth'. It appears to be self-evident that an ethical norm must always have at least one ethical value. Other values that can be an integral part of an ethical norm include *life, freedom, love, happiness, friendship, fidelity, loyalty, fraternity, peace, security, justice, benevolence, truth, trustworthiness*, etc. All of these are regarded as intrinsic values, and therefore they can serve as ends for our actions. In contrast, such items as money, car, house, boat, aeroplane, pen, computer, medicine, etc. are regarded as having only extrinsic or instrumental value. They cannot be ends, but only means to ends – to what has ethically intrinsic value. They gain their extrinsic value from the ends that they are used to achieve. For example, a medicine has instrumental value to the extent that it can promote heath. When it loses its power to do so, it automatically loses its value.

What is a view of life and what is a view of man?

In referring to a *view of life*, we mean the same as a *philosophy of life*, which is an integral part of a worldview, culture, religion, ideology, etc. A view of life can be either religious or profane. Christianity, Judaism and Islam, for example, contain a religious view of the human race. Examples of non-religious views or philosophies of life include humanism, atheistic existentialism (according to, for example, Sartre and Camus), Marxism and certain types of feminism. Each view of life describes and explains human life in its ideal form (when it is at its best) and in its decayed form (when it is at its worst).[18] Thus a humanistic ideal of life comprises, among other things, values such as dignity, freedom, liberty, happiness, security and peace for individuals and groups. Where these values are lacking, life will not flourish, but may assume its worst form. A view of life states some necessary conditions that each individual should fulfil in order to attain the highest ideal of life. For example, Judaism, Christianity and Islam teach that life's highest goal is the individual's fellowship with his or her fellow human beings and with God. On the other hand, Hinduism claims that it is deliverance (in Sanskrit, *nirvana*) from reincarnation (in Sanskrit, *samsara*). A view of life contains a view of the human race, which is closely related to a concept of morality and ethics.[19]

Human dignity according to a humanistic and a non-humanistic view of the human race

The greatest difference between these two views of the human race is that the humanistic view holds that all human beings have the same dignity and worth. In contrast, the non-humanistic view of the human race holds that all human beings do not have equal dignity and worth.* It is noteworthy that whereas humanistic views of the human race emphasise *what* is common to all human beings, non-humanistic views of the human race emphasise the difference between human individuals.

How does a humanistic view of the human race justify human dignity and worth?

The most prominent feature of all humanistic views is that all of them hold that human dignity and worth should be based on the following:

1 intellect (human beings are rational)
2 freedom or autonomy (human beings have free will, freedom of choice and action)
3 goodness (human beings have the potential for goodness, but they are dependent on both heredity and environment).

Classic humanism regards the above three properties as distinctive features of human nature and as the foundation of human dignity and worth. This is, for example, the view of Kant.[20] Classic humanism maintains that all human beings are equal solely on the grounds of human dignity and worth – that is, without the need to fulfil any condition.

All humanistic views of the human race characterise human dignity and worth as *constant, immeasurable or inestimable and non-gradable, unconditional, inalienable* and *inviolable.* The notion that human dignity is *constant* means that it does not increase or decrease with the individual's age, gender, social or health status,

---

* Cf. Article No. 1 in United Nations' Universal Declaration of Human Rights of 10 December 1948.

ethnic origin, capacity, etc. The notion that human dignity is *immeasurable* and *non-gradable* is an aspect of its constancy and means that human dignity is the same for men and women, white and black, king and slave, rich and poor, sick and healthy, free men and prisoners, etc. Thus no one is ethically justified in asking which of two or more individuals has more (or higher) dignity and worth. The notion that human dignity is *unconditional* means that every human being has it solely because he/she is human, without the need or prerequisite to fulfil any other condition. The Universal Declaration of Human Rights, Article 1, declares that everyone is born with the same dignity and worth. To say that human dignity and worth are *inalienable* means that they are not transferable. In other words, an individual's dignity and worth is incapable of being transferred to other people. This is in contrast to a person's autonomy, which is transferable to others (e.g. to parents, advocates, etc.). Finally, the notion that human dignity is *inviolable* means ethically speaking that it should or ought not to be violated. Regrettably, however, it is violated every day worldwide.

For all forms of humanism, human dignity is the ethical foundation of the most basic human rights, such as the right to life, the right to security (or 'happiness') and the right to liberty. The term *liberty* refers to political and civil rights, freedom of thought, freedom of conscience, freedom of expression, freedom of religion, etc. These and other basic human rights are the foundation for other human rights such as the right to school education, the right to healthcare, the right to employment and the right to privacy, as well as economic, social and cultural rights, etc.

It is therefore extremely important to answer the question of what value a human being has, because human value (dignity and worth) is the ethical basis of all human rights. Furthermore, it is the basis of morality and ethics (i.e. how we should treat others and ourselves, how we should behave and what attitude we should have towards one another, to all living beings, and to nature and the environment).

To summarise, we can say that the humanistic view of the human race, as the basis of humanistic ethics, promotes human autonomy, dignity, the basic equality of all human beings and each human being's basic rights, according to the United Nations' Universal Declaration of 1948, supplemented by later conventions on human rights.* This consideration has great relevance in arguing for or against induced abortion.

How does the non-humanistic view of the human race justify human dignity and worth?

As mentioned previously, a non-humanistic view is the opposite of a humanistic one. It therefore denies what the latter affirms, namely the basic equality of all human beings with regard to their dignity and worth, and basic rights. It was also mentioned earlier in this chapter that the non-humanistic view emphasises the differences or inequalities between all human individuals. Thus the non-humanistic view bases the value of each individual on the following criteria:

---

* See *Convention on Human Rights and Biomedicine*. Council of Europe. Directorate of Legal Affairs, Strasbourg 1997.

1 the individual's *utilitarian value* – their value based on their merit or achievement and contribution to public welfare through their own effort
2 the individual's *affective significance*
3 the individual's *moral value* (based on their *moral integrity*). For example, Mother Teresa, Francis of Assisi and Martin Luther King are regarded as having a higher degree of moral integrity than most other people.

The utilitarian value refers to what individuals can accomplish by their own effort, and which promotes the welfare of society or mankind. With regard to the affective significance or value that an individual has for other people, in most cases people are of great affective significance or value to their parents, their children, their partner, their friends, etc. (i.e. significant others), and vice versa. However, there are many people who live alone. Perhaps they have no affective value for anyone. Therefore if the criterion of affective significance is used to assess their value, these people may be found to have no value at all. At any rate they have less value than those who, for example, have parents, friends, etc., according to the non-humanistic view. Furthermore, an assessment of individuals' value according to their utilitarian value leads to a quantification of their value, as a consequence of which they must have different rights, since human rights follow from human value.

To summarise, we can say that the non-humanistic view necessarily implies a quantification of human beings according to the value that they have achieved by means of their own effort. This undermines the equality of all human beings. It therefore has ethical consequences for how one ought to apply, for example, the formal principle of *justice* (defined by Aristotle* as 'equals must be treated equally, and unequals must be treated unequally') in social ethics. From a humanistic point of view, social justice is the application of this formal principle of justice in combination with the principle of equity and fundamental needs as material criteria for distributive justice. From a non-humanistic point of view, in contrast, the concept of social justice is a combination of the formal principle of justice with one or more of the three criteria listed above. Since the non-humanistic view quantifies and discriminates between individuals on the basis of their differences, it has negative consequences for the treatment of marginalised groups in society (e.g. the fetus or zygote, babies, children, elderly people, handicapped and sick people, immigrants, etc.). For further information about the quantification of human beings, the non-humanistic view and its consequences for morality and ethics, the reader is referred to the relevant literature.[21]

Which view of man is the true or proper one?

There is no simple answer to this question. The following reflection may help an individual to find out his or her own personal answer.[22] It seems to be common knowledge that human beings can experience themselves and contemplate themselves both as subjects and objects. To regard oneself as a subject is strictly related to one's experience of oneself (i.e. the experience of one's self-awareness, identity, dignity and worth – the meaning *in* and the meaning *of* one's life and suffering). To look at oneself as an object implies that people can function at the same time as subjects or agents *and* as manipulable objects upon which they, as subjects, can

---

* Beauchamp TL & Childress JF. *Principles of Biomedical Ethics*. Oxford: Oxford University Press, 2001.

reflect and from which they can distance themselves emotionally and intellectually. This can enable us to study both other people and ourselves objectively.

In choosing one view of the human race from among many different ones, in a pluralistic world, it is relevant to consider both the subjective and objective ways of studying a human being. Furthermore, one should argue for and choose the view of the human race that does justice to one's accumulated experiences of what it means to be a human being. These experiences comprise or include one's conception of human life when it is at its best as well as when it is at its worst. Our experience of what it means to be human is dependent on various factors. One such factor is our culture – our knowledge of mankind's accumulated experiences of and our reflection upon the existential question '*What is a human being?*' One obtains different answers to this question from, for example, mythology, literature, art, religion, philosophy and the various sciences.

The relationship between view of life, view of the human race and ethics

It was pointed out earlier, when examples of moral norms and values were given, that a moral norm always contains at least one moral value – as in the example, 'One should tell the truth.' However, one norm may contain several values – for example, 'One should respect a person's *dignity*, *worth* and *autonomy*, and his or her *basic rights* (e.g. his or her right to participate in decisions concerning him or her).' The italicised words denote moral values. One important and relevant question in this context is how the individual develops his or her values. The short answer is that they are obtained from the view of life and the view of the human race that exist in his or her culture or religion, in which he or she grows up and learns to interact with others. From this point of view, moral norms and values may vary from one person to another according to their culture and/or religion. Thus an Indian culture or religion does not contain exactly the same values and norms as those of a Christian, Muslim or Confucian culture. In addition, we can say that an atheist and a religious person do not endorse exactly the same values and norms. However, this fact does not exclude the existence of cross-cultural values – for example, that life, well-being and peace have intrinsic value, and norms such as 'One should tell the truth', 'It is wrong to kill an innocent person' and 'One should help people in need.'[23]

With regard to the ethical problem of abortion, it is a person's view of the human race, gained from within his or her culture or religion, that 'tells' him or her whether or not the *zygote, embryo* and *fetus* have human dignity and worth.

Perhaps the aborting woman's experience of feelings of guilt or emotional ambivalence after an induced abortion wholly or partly depends on her belief that only one true ethical norm exists, with the help of which one can evaluate whether an abortion is ethically right or not.* From the perspective of a holistic approach to the ethical problem of abortion, it is possible to provide better ethical guidance for both the aborting woman and the other agents involved in induced abortions. Another relevant issue where there is a need for guidance is the relationship between what is right according to law and what is ethical and morally right.

---

* She needs the following kind of advice: '*whether the harm, to a women, of carrying an unwanted pregnancy to full term outweighs the harm of undergoing an abortion*'; www.issuesinmedicalethics.org/131di018.html (accessed 14 May 2005).

The concepts of right and wrong according to law and ethics

The main purpose of this section is to emphasise that what is right according to law may be morally wrong, even with regard to abortion. It should be pointed out that rules of law may differ from one country to another, and usually do so. Therefore the fact that, for example, induced abortion is now *legally* right according to Swedish law cannot be inferred as saying anything about whether abortion is also legally right or wrong, or should be legally right, in other countries, or whether or not it always ought to be so.[24] In certain Roman Catholic countries and in Islamic countries, the law prohibits abortion. Thus, taking Europe as an example, even within the European Community the abortion laws differ (compare the law on free abortion in Ireland, Poland, Spain and Portugal). However, the ethical norms 'You shall not kill an innocent person' and 'One should help a person in need' seem to have universal and cross-cultural normative validity. In contrast, rules of law are usually normatively valid in a particular country and over a particular period of time. They impose duties primarily on the citizens of the countries and defend their rights and privileges. With regard to present-day democracies, the relationship between rules of law (RL) and rules of ethics (RE) can be illustrated as shown in Figure 8.2.

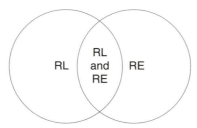

Figure 8.2 The relationship between rules of law and rules of ethics. The area denoted by RL contains the class of actions that are right only according to law. The area denoted by RE contains the class of actions that are right only according to ethics. The common area denoted by RL and RE contains the class of actions that are right according to both law and ethics in the same country.

Although the research studies described in this book show that it is rare for women who have an abortion to experience feelings of guilt, there are a few examples of women experiencing such feelings up to 10 to 20 years after an induced abortion (*see* Chapter 6).[22] This could be explained by the fact that during the decision-making process that led to her choosing an abortion, the woman might have believed that what is right according to the law is always ethically right, at least with regard to abortion, but later on she might have changed her belief.

The handling of the aborted fetus in the light of normative ethics

In Chapter 2 of this book, in the section on the handling of the aborted fetus, it was stated that: 'according to the new recommendations,[25] fetuses from late abortions (spontaneous or induced) from the beginning of week 13 up to and including week 28 should be sent from the maternity clinic to the pathology department. Later the fetus is taken to a crematorium to be cremated, and the ashes are buried or spread anonymously. There is also the possibility of interment or of a burial ceremony if the woman or the couple so wish. In this case the mother and the fetus are no longer anonymous.'

From the viewpoint of the ethics of healthcare, this can be interpreted either positively or negatively. Some aborting women may interpret it positively when an abortion is inevitable and they experience it not only as right according to law, but also as morally right. In this case a funeral of the fetus is welcome, and it may have a positive function in providing a way of grieving, supported by family members and friends. However, if the woman does not experience abortion as both legally and morally right, she may have negative feelings about such a funeral, because it will remind her of a presumptive morally wrong course of action that she took, which cannot be undone, and this can give rise to genuine feelings of guilt.

Furthermore, the cremation or burial of the fetus has a morally suspect aspect because it can affect aborting women negatively, especially those who 'have no need of grieving' for the loss of their fetus, 'are not disposed to grieve' or 'simply do not want to grieve.'[26] For these women the burial ceremony may generate feelings of ambivalence and guilt, regardless of whether they were morally responsible for choosing abortion or not. Their ambivalent feelings may be due to sometimes believing that it was morally right to choose abortion, and sometimes believing that it was morally wrong.

A holistic approach to abortion

The results of the investigation described in this book indicate that the complexity of abortion is not always taken into consideration in the ethical assessment of the various alternative courses of action that are available when arguing for or against abortion. There are many aspects of abortion that are relevant in this context, and therefore they should be emphasised. Some examples include the following:

1 the body of the aborting woman and the biology and physiology of the fetus
2 the health, age and psychological, social, economic and political status of the aborting woman and her partner
3 the ethical, aesthetic, existential and religious dimensions of the abortion.

Under aspect 3 in the above list the factors that should be considered include the responsibility of the abortionists and those who use tissues from the aborted fetus (e.g. for transplantation).[27] During the last 10 to 15 years it is aspects 1 and 2 in the above list that seem to have been most clearly highlighted by the aborting woman's decision making about abortion, which led to her choice to terminate her pregnancy.

Instead a holistic approach to abortion that also takes into consideration aspect 3 is suggested here. Such an approach would involve an analysis and assessment of abortion in the light of all three above-mentioned aspects. A holistic approach has the following advantages.

First, it means that not all of the responsibility for the choice of an abortion has to be attributed to the aborting woman. Several agents may share with her the responsibility for her choice of abortion. These may include her partner and/or his parents, the society in which she lives, the abortionists and her own parents. None of them should be reduced to a simple means of carrying out the apparently mechanical or routine action of inducing an abortion, without any personal engagement in and moral responsibility for what they do.[28]

Secondly, a holistic approach allows openness in the ethical assessment of individual cases, so that each aborting woman's unique situation and needs can be taken into consideration. This means that not only her economic status but also other features of her situation and identity should be taken into account (e.g. her health status and religious beliefs).[22]

In Sweden a pregnant woman is no longer obliged to ask for assistance from a counselling board if her pregnancy is within the first 12 weeks. Nevertheless, as our interviews with psychiatrists and Catholic priests demonstrate, many pregnant and aborting women need help and/or support with regard to aspect 3 listed above, especially the ethical, existential and religious dimensions. At least the abortionists – as healthcare professionals – have a moral obligation to respect the aborting woman's autonomy, which in this context should be interpreted both as her right to self-determination and as her right to participate in all decision making about her interests.[29] To use the latter right, she should be well informed about the different courses of action available and their respective possible consequences for her both in the short term and in the long term. Accordingly, in dealing with abortion from a holistic point of view, we should obey the Swedish Health and Social Law of 1982 (HSL 82), which states that good health and social care should be based on patients' right to respect for their dignity and worth and to participate in decision making about their care.[30]

Summary and concluding remarks

This chapter has provided an ethical reflection on the problem of free abortion and on various factors leading to the inducement of abortion. It has indicated that the book as a whole aims to demonstrate the complexity of abortion – that is, its many different aspects, and the fact that it involves several agents in addition to the aborting woman as the central agent. The various aspects of abortion concern and engage the aborting woman, her partner and perhaps her parents, the society in which she lives, the abortionists and the healthcare system. Therefore, in attributing moral responsibility for a case of free abortion, one should take into consideration the extent to which each of these agents is implicated. Thus one should not attribute all of the responsibility for the decision to have an abortion to the aborting woman, even if she is the main agent by virtue of the fact that she is the only person to whom the law of free abortion gives the ultimate right to decide whether to undergo induced abortion or not.

Furthermore, it is suggested that a just distribution of moral responsibility among the various agents mentioned above requires a holistic approach to abortion, which seriously considers the legal, political, economic, physiological, psychological, existential, aesthetic, ethical and religious dimensions of abortion. This holistic requirement seems to be reasonable in a pluralistic society with respect to views of life and concepts of the human race, and a democratic society, the basic values of which (e.g. equality and the right to social justice for all citizens) have their anthropological basis, *inter alia*, in a humanistic view of human life.

References

1 Kuhse H. *Caring: women and ethics* (Swedish text). Oxford: Blackwell Publishers, 1997.

2 Mathewes-Green F. Why women choose abortion. Post-abortion interviews reveal what would have changed their minds. *Christianity Today.* 1995; 9 January: 21–5. See also Moreau C, Kaminski M, Ancel PY *et al.* Previous induced abortions and the risk of very preterm delivery: results of the EPIPAGE study. *Int J Obstet Gynecol.* 2005; **112:** 430–37.

3 Sherwin S. Abortion: a feminist perspective. In: JD Arras & B Steinbock (eds) *Ethical Issues in Modern Medicine.* Mountain View, CA: Mayfield Publishing Company, 1999. See also Callahan S. A case for pro-life-feminism. In: JD Arras & B Steinbock (eds) *Ethical Issues in Modern Medicine.* Mountain View, CA: Mayfield Publishing Company, 1999.

4 Thunberg A-M. The social dimensions of abortion (Swedish text). In: C-H Grenholm *et al.* (eds) *Etiska Texter [Ethical Texts].* Lund: Verbum Håkan Ohlssons, 1977.

5 Kant identifies free will or autonomy with 'practical reason.' Cf. Heubel F & Biller-Andorno N. The contribution of Kantian moral theory to contemporary medical ethics: a critical analysis. *Med Healthcare Philos.* 2005; **7:** 5–18.

6 Ofstad H. *Responsibility and Action. Introduction to moral philosophical problems* (Swedish text). Stockholm: Prisma, 1982. Cf. Ofstad H. *An Inquiry into the Freedom of Decision.* Norway: Norwegian University Press, 1961, London: George Allen and Unwin Ltd. In Ofstad's opinion, *freedom of decision* or *action* can be defined as follows: 'P had it in his power to decide D2, instead of D1.' Thus a person is responsible for an action D2 if, and only if, he or she is able to perform D2 or to refrain from performing D2 (ibid 1961: 203). For an account of the way in which freedom, responsibility and moral conscience are related to one another, see Viktor F. *The Unconscious God. Psychotherapy and Religion* (Swedish text). Stockholm: Natur och Kultur, 1987.

7 Mathewes-Green F. Why women choose abortion. Post-abortion interviews reveal what would have changed their minds. *Christianity Today.* 1995; 9 January: 22. Cf. Moreau C. Previous induced abortions and the risk of very preterm delivery: results of the EPIPAGE study. *Int J Obstet Gynaecol.* 2005; **112:** 430.

8 Furberg M. *The First Stone. A moral phenomenological study* (Swedish text). Göteborg: Daidalos, 1999.

9 May R. *The Discovery of Being. Writings in existential psychology.* New York: WW Norton & Company, 1983: 116. Cf. Blomquist C. *Soul and Mind* (Swedish text). Stockholm: Natur och Kultur, 1974.

10 The Roman Catholic Church's view of abortion. A statement of the Nordic Catholic Bishops. In: L Ejerfeldt & H Seiler (eds) *Law and Ethics on the Issue of Abortion* (Swedish text). Stockholm: Credo Katolsk Tidskrift, 1972.

11 Lübcke P (ed.). *Filosofilexikonet [The Dictionary of Philosophy].* Stockholm: Forum, 1994. See also Gert B Hobbes, Thomas. In: *The Cambridge Dictionary of Philosophy.* Cambridge: Cambridge University Press, 1995: 367–70. Hobbes has the same understanding as Plato concerning the role of reason and emotions in ethics.

12 Barbosa da Silva A & Ljungquist M. *Ethics in Healthcare. A moral philosophical analysis of the relationship between views of life, views of man and the concept of illness in an*

historical and systematic perspective (Norwegian text). Stavanger: MHS Förlaget, 2002. See also Nystedt H. *Duty and Love: studies in Nygren's ethics* (Swedish text). Stockholm: Svenska kyrkans diakonistyrelses förlag, 1951.

13 Frankena WK. *Ethics.* Englewood Cliffs, NJ: Prentice-Hall, Inc., 1973. See also Childress TL & Childress JF. *Principles of Biomedical Ethics* (5e). New York: Oxford University Press, 2001.

14 Tännsjö T. *To Produce Children: a study in the ethics of reproductive technology* (Swedish text). Stockholm: Sesan, 1991. Cf. Sundström P. *Abortion in a New Light* (Swedish text). Nora: Nya Doxa, 1994.

15 Herrmann E. *Scientific Theory and Religious Belief. An essay on the rationality of views of life.* Kampen, The Netherlands: Pharos, 1995.

16 Landgren M. Worldview and view of man in changing process (Swedish text). In: T Seidal (ed.) *Human Dignity in Devaluation: ethics at the beginning and at the end of life* (Swedish text). Uppsala: EFS Förlaget, 1986.

17 Hermerén G. *What is Medical Ethics?* In: *Ethics – Responsibility – Communication: Swedish medical corporation and Örebro's medical corporation's postgraduate training course* (Swedish text). Stockholm: SPRI, 1984: 7–16.

18 Cf. Herrmann E. God, reality and the religious philosophical debate about realism and anti-realism (Swedish text). *STK.* 1999; **75:** 51–63. See also Herrmann E. *Scientific Theory and Religious Belief. An essay on the rationality of views of life.* Kampen, The Netherlands: Pharos, 1995.

19 Grenholm C-H, Holte R, Hemberg J *et al. Ethical Problems* (Swedish text). Lund: Verbum Håkan Ohlssons, 1977.

20 Bischofberger E. From human dignity to human rights. In: *The Diffuseness of the Concept of Human Dignity: a debate paper. Ethical Signposts 4* (Swedish text). Stockholm: Statens medicinsk-etiska råd, 1993.

21 Barbosa da Silva A. The value and meaning of the human life before and after birth. (Swedish text). *Svensk tidskrift foniatri logopedi.* 1988; **1:** 4–11.

22 Most of the argument presented in this section is taken from Barbosa da Silva A & Andersson M. *Science and Views of Man in Healthcare. An introduction to the philosophy of science and healthcare ethics* (Swedish text). Stockholm: SHSTF, 1993, 1996. See also Barbosa da Silva A & Ljungquist M. *Ethics in Healthcare. A moral philosophical analysis of the relationship between views of life, views of man and the concept of illness in an historical and systematic perspective* (Norwegian text). Stavanger: MHS Förlaget, 2002. Cf. Holte R. *Man's Interpretation of Life and Belief in God. Theories and methods within the sciences of religious belief and view of life* (Swedish text). Lund: Doxa, 1984.

23 Cf. Barbosa da Silva A and Ljungquist M. *Healthcare Ethics for a Multicultural Sweden. A theoretical and empirical analysis of some necessary conditions for open and holistic healthcare in a pluralistic society* (Swedish text). Lund: Studentlitteratur, 2003.

24 Ofstad H. *Our Contempt for Human Weakness. An analysis of the Nazis' norms and values* (Swedish text). Oslo: Pax, 1991. Cf. Sundström P. *Abortion in a New Light* (Swedish text). Nora: Nya Doxa, 1994. See also Dworkin R. *Taking Rights Seriously.* London: Duckworth, 1978. Hemberg J. *Ethics and Legislation. A study of theory construction within philosophy of law and concrete legislation work* (Swedish text). Stockholm: Verbum-Dialog, 1975.

25 National Board of Health and Welfare. *General Advice Regarding the Disposal of Aborted Fetuses* (Swedish text). Stockholm: National Board of Health and Welfare, 1990.

26 Stenius Y. Abortion ... and the man that wants to deliver us from our moral conscience (Swedish text). *Aftonbladet.* 1990; 11 November: 4–5. See also Mathewes-Green F. Why women choose abortion. Post-abortion interviews

reveal what would have changed their minds. *Christianity Today.* 1995; 9 January: 21–5. Ofstad H. *Our Contempt for Human Weakness. An analysis of the Nazis' norms and values* (Swedish text). Oslo: Pax, 1991. Sundström P. *Abortion in a New Light* (Swedish text). Nora: Nya Doxa, 1994. Dworkin R. *Taking Rights Seriously.* London: Duckworth, 1978.

27 Sundström P. *Abortion in a New Light* (Swedish text). Nora: Nya Doxa, 1994.

28 Bischofberger E & Brattgård H. The inviolable human dignity. In: *The Diffuseness of the Concept of Human Dignity: a debate paper. Ethical Signposts 4.* Stockholm: Statens medicinsk-etiska råd, 1993.

29 Tranøy KE. *Medical Ethics Today* (Swedish text). Lund: Studentlitteratur, 1991.

30 Andersson M. *Dignity as a Concept and as an Ethical Principle. A study of an ideal healthcare ethics in development* (Swedish text). Finland: Åbo Akademi, 1996.

Chapter 9

Personal reflections by the editor

Vivian Wahlberg

Introduction

My own background

During the many years I have been practising my profession, first for a short period as a school nurse, then for several years as a midwife, and later as a researcher, I have met many young people with widely varying thoughts, feelings and experiences. They have told me about complicated situations, struggles with their own body image, unhappy love affairs, contraception, and their search for solutions to difficult teenage problems. Later in life they sometimes describe feelings of confusion and sorrow about an unwanted pregnancy. I have met many young people facing an abortion, as mentioned earlier in this book, but I have also seen young people in love and experiencing joy about a pregnancy – when a new human life is on the way.

As a midwife I have been responsible for more than a thousand deliveries, and in each case I have been at the woman's side during one of the most unique moments of life, and have tried to give the new family the help that they needed at this time. In addition, as part of my study for a degree in sociology, I studied the adoption process by following up around 250 couples with regard to their longing for and plans to adopt a child.

All of this provided a varied and comprehensive background to my last 25 years of research and teaching in the field of caring and public health. These last years have involved projects not only in Sweden but also in many other countries worldwide, which have given me further insight into the differences in the experience of birth and death in poor and more developed parts of the world.

A contrast to our modern age

As a contrast to our modern way of life, I often think about a small booklet[1] that presents the biography of a family over four generations, starting nearly 150 years ago.

Falling in love, getting engaged, and family circumstances in the nineteenth century and well into the twentieth century were quite different from the situation today. Just as society has undergone major changes in other respects, so the patterns of relationships and married life have also changed. Today we have a considerably more open and natural view of sexuality and how it can be used as a positive resource between two people.

The story of Gotland House

From the middle of the nineteenth century

In order to give some idea of how life has varied in different eras, I want to give a short review of how earlier generations experienced their life and housing, as described in the above-mentioned booklet, *Gotland House,* from the mid-nineteenth century.[1] The booklet reflects a time of poverty, difficulties and fears that are unfamiliar to the 'normal' Swedish family of today.

Gotland House is the story of an old farmhouse constructed of greyish-white limestone, reflecting old traditions and having considerable beauty. However, it also describes the extreme poverty, coldness and damp, the wet clothes, the fleas in the rag-carpet, and old people with rounded shoulders, frequent illness and a constant fear of tuberculosis. In addition, the women had a constant fear of becoming pregnant.

The storyteller is a district nurse and midwife who had worked on Gotland, the largest Swedish island, since the mid-twentieth century, and who had met people who were born in the previous century and sat down with them in their old everyday environment, in Gotland House.

The house is situated in a meadow with a mixture of hazel, oak, mountain ash and birch trees. It is an ordinary Gotland house, with one room on either side of the entrance, deep window recesses and heavy ceiling beams. Further details about the house are given:[1]

> The room straight ahead is sometimes used as a guest room and sometimes used for funerals and weddings. At funerals there is a smell of juniper. The room is draped in white for the occasion, and the deceased is dressed and placed on a bier, to give neighbours and friends an opportunity to say goodbye for the last time. When it is time for a wedding celebration, the bride is dressed for her wedding in this room ... At wedding festivities the front garden is decorated with a triumphal arch, a 'young man pole' and young birch trees. At the top of the house there is a special room where the old people spend their last years.

The story describes the hard life of the people who lived in the house and toiled from early morning until late at night. It was a life characterised by fear, anger and poverty. Life was hard on these people, but they were also hard on each other. The booklet describes how the married life of the husband and wife, born in 1866 and 1873, respectively, was shrouded in mystery and taboo. It was a time when male domination was the rule, and the man had the authority to own both his wife and his property. It is a narrative about silence, bitterness and rape within marriage, and about the woman's constant fear of becoming pregnant.

Throughout pregnancy, the woman was to be kept under lock and key – she was not allowed to be seen to be pregnant, as this was regarded as something unsightly. The old Christian idea prevailed that she had become unclean during sexual intercourse with her husband and remained unclean during the pregnancy and until six weeks after the delivery, when she had to be 'registered' in the church again (in order to be re-accepted into the church community). Through this act she would be forgiven for having agreed to have intercourse with her clean husband. The child was also regarded as unclean until he or she had been baptised.[1]

A positive change over time

The story of Gotland House is not just a tale of tragic conditions in earlier generations. It also deals with an enormous positive change over time, and describes how life for children, grandchildren and great-grandchildren altered and improved little by little, and how the sex life of the later generations began to be characterised by mutual respect and closeness. Contraceptives were now available, and falling in love and the expression of passionate feelings were now accepted. Sexuality and its consequences, which had been a heavy burden for many earlier generations, were now characterised by attitudes of openness and longing. Love and sexuality were now experienced as a legitimate source of pleasure and satisfaction.

Love as a mainstay of strength

Throughout human history, it has been documented in philosophy, religion, literature and elsewhere how human beings need to be loved and also to share their love with other people. Love is a mainstay of strength both in everyday life and on special occasions. Love is a resource for the purpose of creating life through our sexual drive. Most often conception that results in a new life occurs in a context of love and passion. However, love is also a resource during life and for the further progression of life. Sigmund Freud (1856–1939), the famous psychiatrist and founder of psychoanalysis, spoke of the deep structure of love and stated that in a love relationship one loves the other person because one finds a positive picture of oneself in him or her. Moreover, Freud said that love is a healing process. In a love relationship the psyche is an open system that is associated with and dependent on the other person.

A notable article entitled 'A psychoanalytical meditation on marriage'[2] sheds light on different aspects of marriage as a process, which can result in either disappointment and bitterness or unity and personal maturity. Truly unselfish love leads ultimately to personal development. In a section on mirroring, the author points out the lifelong ambition of individuals to be seen as the people that they are, and to be able to be themselves – that is, we as individuals want to be the people that we were created to be. To be ourselves we need confirmation by other people. In our relationships with other people, we confirm or deny one another – that is, mirroring takes place. The question is whether it is the right picture that is reflected. Is the opposite party just and honest, upright and truthful?

A mirror can be ground and clear and give a 'true image', or it can be cloudy and give a blurred and 'foggy' image, or it can be uneven and give a distorted image.[2] In mutual mirroring an intimate and trustful closeness is established, which ideally the partners can express both mentally and physically in their sexual relationship. This is just what a person requires in order to feel needed and loved! However, confidence and sincerity in a relationship require commitment and hard work, with a constant effort to give and take in a genuine encounter.

Self-knowledge and maturity

There was little justice in life a century ago, but neither is it easy today. Now and then most of us experience feelings of ambivalence, particularly when we are facing decisions of vital importance, such as the question of whether to have an abortion.

People can sometimes experience a threat to their very existence, their social identity and sense of security and their aims in life. At such times they may try to keep reality at a distance. However, it is vitally important to try to get help and to express in words the traumatic and difficult feelings. When facing the question of abortion, talking about one's feelings has a therapeutic effect and is part of the decision-making process and later the adaptation process.

It is not only the concrete, obvious questions that are of decisive importance in determining how one feels and acts in a particular situation. Each person has within them deep, intangible experiences and thoughts that can influence their feelings and actions. These may be experiences from childhood, thoughts associated with earlier relationships, or a lack of confidence in life. However, perhaps one's earlier experience of life is not enough to enable one to handle the current situation. The way in which that situation should be solved will depend on the life circumstances as well as the personality of each individual. The present is always more important than the past, as is demonstrated by the narratives presented in this book about young women's and men's thoughts, feelings and experiences of sorrow and confusion, all layered with dreams and visions of the future.

It is said that self-knowledge and maturity increase over the years, but in the autumn of my life I am still asking myself the same questions that are raised by many young people on the threshold of adulthood:

Who am I? Where do I come from? And where am I going?

References

1 Olsson H. *Gotlandshuset – Gotland House (the story of B Larsson)* (Swedish text). Stockholm: National Board of Health and Welfare, 1978.
2 Basch-Kåhre E. A psychoanalytical meditation on marriage (Swedish text). *Signum.* 1992; **18**(9): 286–90.

Index

3